The TROUBLE *with* MEDICINE

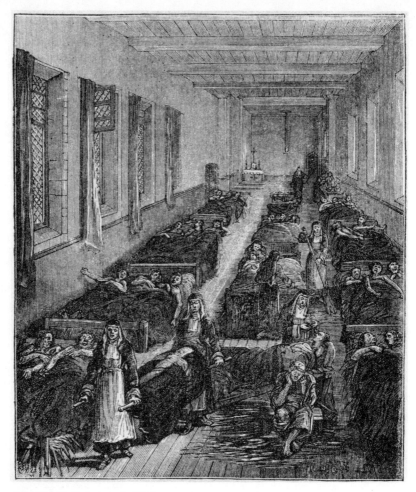

Ward in Paris hospital, 1718

The
TROUBLE
with
MEDICINE

D R M E L V I N K O N N E R

BBC BOOKS

PICTURE CREDITS

BBC Books would like to thank the following for providing photographs, and for permission to reproduce copyright material. While every effort has been made to trace and acknowledge all copyright holders, we would like to apologize should there have been any errors or omissions:

1 Lisa Laurie; 2 Rosie Allsop; 3 Rosie Allsop; 4 Rosie Allsop; 5 Lisa Laurie; 6 Alex Hansen; 7 Alex Hansen; 8 Ron Foley; 9 Ron Foley; 10 Ron Foley; 11 Claire Broughton; 12 The Cleveland Clinic; 13 Kerry Herman; 14 Rosie Allsop; 15 David South; 16 David South; 17 Martin Patmore; 18 Rajish Bedi; 19 Rajish Bedi; 20 Ron Foley; 21 Sandy Edwards

ISBN 0 563 36377 0

Designed by David Robinson

First published in hardback by BBC Books,
a division of BBC Enterprises Limited
Woodlands, 80 Wood Lane, London W12 0TT

First published in 1993

Set in Bembo by Selwood Systems, Midsomer Norton
Colour separations by Dot Gradations Ltd, South Woodham Ferrers, near Chelmsford
Jacket printed by Lawrence Allen Ltd, Weston-super-Mare
Printed and bound in Great Britain by Butler & Tanner, Frome and London

CONTENTS

ACKNOWLEDGEMENTS

In a project of this kind, the author has an unusual range and degree of indebtedness. To say that this book would not have been possible without the help of *The Trouble with Medicine* television series production team is to put the matter mildly. Their enormous talent and long, hard work have formed the structure and substance of the remarkable materials at my disposal in writing this book. While they generously assure me that some of my own knowledge and ideas have found a way into their films, and while they bear little or no responsibility for any errors in my book, I know that my debt to them is far greater than theirs to me.

The series is a co-production of BBC Science and Features Department, the PBS station Thirteen/WNET, New York, the Australian Broadcasting Company, Sydney, and TV Española. I thank Martin Freeth and Stefan Moore, co-executive producers of the series, who oriented me to the project, read my entire manuscript twice, and provided extensive criticism and discussion. Freeth was also producer-director of episode three, 'The Magic Bullet', and Moore was producer-director of 'Temple of Science' and co-producer-director of 'Pandemic'. Their contributions to the corresponding chapters were especially great.

Producer-directors of individual episodes were also exceptionally generous with their time and criticism: Stephen White ('Code of Silence'); Jane West ('Random Cuts'); Peter Montagnon ('Disordered States'); Henry Singer ('Life Support'); Tim Clark ('Conceiving the Future'); and Susan Lambert ('Pandemic'). Michele Renay, Kate Akerman and Catherine Drew served as coordinators between the book and the films from the British end, as did Kerry Herman and David Wolff from the American end. Jack Sameth and George Page, production executives at WNET, also helped facilitate the book's development; Carlos Martinez Ramos, Iñigo Yrizar, Luis Agudo and Paco Garrido Lonzano represented TV Española. Patients, physicians and other health workers, and health authorities around the world consented to be filmed and interviewed. Many found their way into this book and are named as they appear; others influenced the text indirectly. I thank them all for their generosity with time and knowledge.

David Wolff, WNET's book editor, was responsible for arranging my participation in the project, and has since provided much welcome support and encouragement. My agent, Elaine Markson, and her capable staff were also crucial to these arrangements. At BBC Books, Heather Holden-Brown provided support and encouragement at the outset. Martha Caute, the book's supervising editor, has worked hard and patiently while I imposed one delay after another on a very tight schedule; her tolerant enthusiasm for the project has been invaluable. Ann Wilson is one of the best copy-editors I have worked with, and both I and my readers owe her a great debt. Christine Shuttleworth prepared the index.

My research assistant, Nancy Lee, provided extensive and capable help specific to the book; David Reisman at WNET provided additional assistance at crucial junctures. Kate Akerman, Rosie Allsop, Sunita Berry, Terence Bradley, Jennifer Crone, Catherine Drew, Evonne Francis and Michele Renay at BBC Science and Features provided both background research for the series, without which the book would not have been possible, and specific research for the book when that was needed. I am grateful. Kate Akerman did the photo research for the book.

Advisors to the series were indirectly advisors to the book whether or not I personally consulted with them. I was able to read not only their published writings but also unpublished ones, as well as transcripts of conversations during advisory meetings that took place before I joined the project. Although they are not in any way responsible for my views, their own are fundamental to the book. They include Doctors Christine Cassel, David Eddy, Harvey Fineberg, Cecil Helman, Anne Kern, Arthur Kleinman, George Lundberg, Roy Porter, Octavi Quintana Trias, Frederick Robbins, Wendy Savage, Victor Sidel, Mary Tudor Hart and John Wennberg, as well as Jean Robinson of the Patients' Association/General Medical Council.

Among the advisors, Doctors Julian Tudor Hart and William Foege must be singled out for exceptional generosity in consulting with me directly. Others who shared their expertise include Doctors Henry Kahn, Boyd Eaton, Sally McNagny, John Stone, Herbert Karp, Ian McColl, Steven Cohen-Cole, Mark Rosenberg, Margaret Mermin, Stuart Seidman, Timothy Harlan, Sir Walter Bodmer and Jennifer Weil, and Professors Carol Worthman, Wenda Trevathan, James Gustafson, Robert Hahn, Fred Kroger and Paul Starr. The manuscript was read in its entirety by Doctors Roger Larsen, Ira Schwartz and Julian Gomez, and Professor Peter Brown. Their comments were invaluable.

The Department of Anthropology and the administration of Emory University were generous in accepting the burden of my absence on short notice for a full academic year. I particularly thank Professors Peter Brown and Peggy Barlett, President James T. Laney and Provost William Frye. Anthropology department staff members Judy Robertson, Shirley Sabo, and Anne Nugent were helpful in facilitating my work on the book while I was on leave.

Early influences on my idea of what a doctor is shaped the consciousness that underlies this book. They include our local general practitioner in Brooklyn, New York, Milton Finkel, my uncle Abraham ('Bobby') Fink and my cousins Leon Fink and Martin Silbersweig – all dedicated primary care doctors. Doctors Paul Pavel, Stefan Stein and Julian Gomez all encouraged and guided my strange career in medicine at crucial junctures. Teachers who played a great role in my medical education are Doctors Hans Bode, Joseph Lipinski, Walter Abelmann, T. Berry Brazelton, Norman Geschwind, Daniel Federman, Edward Gross, Ross Neisuler, Thomas Ballantine, David Hamburg, Francis Moore and Leon Eisenberg. Doctors John Stone, Herbert Karp and Boyd Eaton have been influential models, as well as friends, in the time since. Participation in a seminar at the Center for Advanced Study in the Behavioral Sciences during 1986–87, with Doctors Lawrence Crowley, P. Herbert Leiderman, Robert Rose and Albert Rothenberg, and Professors Robert Scott and Julius Moravcik, helped me to see that my doubts about the way medicine is practised are often shared by others more experienced than I.

Joseph Beck and Dudley Clendinen have been valued advisors and friends. Robert Liebman provided supportive friendship as well as an insight into the British health care system. My brother, Larry Konner, is also my closest friend; we have weathered many trials together, including major illnesses. The same is true of my wife, Marjorie Shostak; her support for my work on this book during a difficult time in her own life has been crucial indeed. Finally, my children, Susanna, Adam and Sarah, are now all old enough to understand what goes into making a book, what this one's purposes are, and what my preoccupation with it may have cost them. Their generosity has been both informed and real, and I am both apologetic and grateful.

INTRODUCTION

When Martin Freeth and Stefan Moore, executive producers of the BBC's *The Trouble With Medicine* series, asked me to write a companion book, it seemed a match made in heaven. My interest had already been aroused when I had heard about the project from David Wolff, the book editor at Thirteen WNET, the American television station co-producing the series. After reading the outline it was clear that Freeth and Moore saw the problems facing modern medicine very similarly to the way I did, which was not entirely surprising since some of the physicians in Britain and the States who were advisors to the series were also among my long-standing heroes.

By working with Freeth and Moore I would be able to draw on material about the practice of medicine around the world, an international approach that particularly attracted me, since I am an anthropologist as well as a (non-practising) physician. The idea was not to produce another series and book on policy, full of dry arguments and drier statistics, but rather to show how policy works itself out on the front line where doctors and other health care workers must carry it out for better or for worse. Among the countries and subjects finally included are a large city hospital and a small town general practice in Japan; mental hospitals in Siena and Rome, and a genetic disease prevention programme in Sardinia; a shop-front counselling centre for pregnant women in Bremen, Germany, and a transforming cardiological practice in East Berlin in the wake of German unification; certain drug- and prostitution-ridden streets of Sydney, Australia; home care health services in Clifden, a seaside village in Galway, Ireland; a general practice in Jarrow, an industrial town in the northeast of England; care of the mentally ill and the dying in the holy city of Benares, India; an AIDS clinic in Bangkok, as well as a rural brothel in Thailand; and hospitals and clinics in many locations in the United States.

The American material illustrates how things can go wrong with modern medicine anywhere, and may well serve as a warning to Britain and other nations suffering from incipient versions of American troubles. While leading British and US government officials frequently claim that America has the best health care in the world, such claims are quite unfounded. On the contrary, health care in the US is in disarray compared with that in Britain and other industrial countries. Fortunately, some features of the American system are unique or almost so; others, however, represent exaggerations of trends that may be seen in lesser forms in Britain and elsewhere.

These include the trend towards rapidly rising costs; increasing specialization at the expense of primary care, in a way that is uncorrelated, or even inversely correlated, with need; increasing emphasis on high-technology medicine, adopted on a wave of enthusiasm and often in the absence of scientific evidence; and a universal tendency to postpone intervention to the acute crisis stage of an illness, rather than taking steps to prevent worsening of the condition at an early stage, or even before the onset of the disease process. These trends, advanced in America, are coming to Britain and elsewhere; the citizens of any country ignore them at their peril.

Although the television series and the book will anger some in the medical profession around the world, both have been prepared with the advice of some of the leading physicians working today. In the book, I have tried to rely on my own authority as little as possible, referring wherever I can to much greater authorities in specialized fields, who are usually named. These, to my mind, enlightened doctors are in a minority in the medical profession at the moment, but I believe that theirs is the voice of the future.

Inevitably, however, the book draws heavily, although usually not explicitly, on my own experience, so it seems appropriate that I should outline what that is. I started out as an anthropologist interested in the interplay between anthropology and medicine. As a young man I spent two years among the Bushmen of the Kalahari Desert in Botswana, doing research for my thesis, and I was struck by their success in coping psychologically with illness and death, without the shields and weapons we consider essential. I even became an apprentice healer in their medicine-trance ceremony – a powerful ritual that mobilizes the creative efforts of an entire village to give spiritual support to an ill person. This experience in Africa confirmed my belief that there is more to healing than the mechanical fixing of physical things that have gone wrong.

After some years as an anthropology professor, I decided to enter medical school. Although I did not end up practising medicine for a living, I experienced first hand the trials and tribulations of medical education, and would later write a book about it. At the same time, I got to know a little of what it feels like to be a doctor – to try to help patients in pain and suffering, suddenly wounded or chronically ill, giving birth or dying; whether they are calm or openly distressed, stoical or defiant, they are almost always confused and fearful – and counting on the doctor to do something clever to put them right.

However critical I have been of doctors – in this book and elsewhere – nothing can erase my basic sympathy for the difficulties, moral, intellectual and practical, that doctors live with every hour of every day. I hope that this sympathy, and the attitudes and policies it leads to, has as clear a place in this book as do the criticisms.

In fact, criticizing doctors, individually or collectively, is not the point. The trouble with medicine today is not trouble with doctors *per se* but rather trouble with a vast social and cultural system. What matters is not pointing a finger of blame, but analysing a system – a society and culture of medicine that has been produced by advanced industrial states. One of the reviews of my book on medical education was called 'The Tribe that Wears White', which names part but by no means all of the problem.

The tribe under study in *The Trouble with Medicine* is all of us – doctors, nurses, hospital administrators, government or insurance company health bureaucrats, malpractice lawyers, pharmaceutical and medical instrument company executives and salespeople, advertisers and public relations representatives for drugs, medical technology, hospitals – and perhaps, above all, patients. The last category sooner or later includes all the others mentioned, plus everyone else in industrial society. And patients are centrally involved in all that happens in medical systems, for good or ill.

It is therefore not irrelevant to mention my own experiences as a patient and as a relative of patients over the past few years. About five years ago my brother's wife had a rare type of major stroke in her brain stem at the age of forty-four; I was involved in her care, which was long and complex, including everything from major surgery to alternative rehabilitative medicine. Ultimately her improvements were great and are still ongoing. Less than a year later my wife began her battle with cancer, so far quite successful, but also long and difficult. Two years after that my mother, at eighty, was drastically incapacitated by a stroke; by the time of her death three months later I had had a new kind of education about the medical care of the elderly and the allocation of resources to the dying.

Then my own long-standing illness, disc problems in the lower back, reached a stage at which even weeks of complete bed rest, which had worked for me when I was younger, could not resolve an acute crisis. I had surgery for repair of two ruptured discs, followed by a long convalescence. Although I was familiar with chronic pain, the new level of pain I experienced then served as another kind of education. And my own central role in maintaining the health of my lower back in future, through exercise and other preventive care, has made my theorizing about prevention very practical and real.

There were other, less dangerous but no less informative experiences. Last year my four-year-old daughter was bitten by a poisonous snake while her mother was out of the country, and I stayed with her in hospital around the clock for a week that included two operations. I had attended her delivery and those of her brother and sister; and while a man can only understand so much and no more about birth, this experience, and delivering thirty-five babies while in medical school, gave me at least a feeling for how crucial is this moment of life. Two of my children were delivered by midwives, an unusual choice in America, and reached by my wife and me after long, hard thought about questions relating to the 'medicalization' of pregnancy and childbirth. Perhaps too, my parents' lifelong deafness made me sensitive from an early age to the conundrums of illness and handicap. And of course, I have had the usual basic education in paediatrics that all involved parents get as their children grow.

At the time of writing this my eighty-one-year-old father is ailing with three moderately serious illnesses – mild heart failure, early stage bladder cancer and intestinal ulcers. He is active and independent, and ideally none of these things should become life-threatening any time soon. But he is (and wants to stay) in a typical American community for the elderly in Florida – something like Sun City, Arizona, described in Chapter 7 – with a series of medical specialists who look at organs instead of the person, and no one doctor who is really paying attention to the whole picture. I had been struck by watching extensive films about Clifden, Ireland, which is contrasted with Sun City in the book and series. There, home visits by non-specialized care givers, and a general practitioner who knows the patient, not just the illnesses, make all the difference in keeping infirm older people alive and independent. So following their lead (a step backward in time and tradition, but a needed one), I have arranged for a visiting nurse to come to my father's home twice a week, and for a physician practising general medicine to give my father the overall medical supervision that he was not getting from the specialists. They will pick up problems before they become crises, and in the end will save the system money. I expect this low-tech 'Irish' approach will work quite well even in Florida, and will extend my father's active life considerably.

I have not recounted this history to impress the reader with my personal medical suffering – indeed, I have been lucky, since most of these experiences have so far ended favourably – but in order to make it clear that I am personally acquainted with the things I am writing about. What follows in these pages may sometimes seem quite abstract and objective, which is as it must be in the final analysis, but behind the abstractions are my subjective experiences of some fairly serious illnesses – all with the accompanying indignities, confusion, cost, fear and pain. I know what it means to be on both sides of the stethoscope.

I do not, certainly, have all the answers, but in this book I have tried to raise some of the most important questions, drawing on my training and experience both professional and personal, and greatly aided by the producers, directors, advisors and others involved in *The Trouble with Medicine*.

To summarize my conclusions briefly – and I think I speak for some others as well – I prefer personal medicine to the impersonal kind that has become common; low-tech primary care to high-tech specialized care wherever that is safely possible (more often than is thought); prevention and early intervention to late-stage crisis management; patient and family involvement in decision-making to medical authoritarianism; a dignified death a little sooner to an over-medicalized one later; a true system of doctor accountability to chaotic malpractice litigation; careful measurement of the outcomes of medical and surgical procedures to the present haphazard system of trial and error; rational and continuous monitoring of the health of a population and active encouragement of early treatment and prevention to the passive stance of a medical system that waits for an illness to present itself; not-for-profit medicine to the cash-register variety; and universal health insurance to the ragged health safety net that exists in the United States.

I fail to see any positive role for private insurance companies in providing that safety net, and would prefer to see a health system more like the Canadian or British one – but with higher funding to bring the underserved up to par – become the model for health care in the United States and elsewhere in the industrial world. There are, however, problems that transcend national boundaries. Surgical operations and diagnostic procedures are subject to inadequate evaluation almost everywhere. Drug companies hawk their wares using methods that typically obfuscate, rather than clarify, the choices that are best for patients. Prevention is pitifully neglected. Doctors and patients alike wait till illness has reached an advanced stage and then look for a quick fix – one that can often cost a fortune and still not work. Almost all of us overestimate what modern medicine can do, and few of us are prepared to face a fact that people in past generations simply could not ignore: all of us must die some time, and if in the process we consume too many of the resources of those who will go on living, we may deny them the kinds of lives we ourselves have had.

Medical training is increasingly biased against primary care and general practice, against prevention and early intervention, against the simplest tactics of nutrition and exercise, immunization and monitoring, house calls and home help. Unnecessary operations by the tens of thousands, including Caesarian sections, pacemaker implantations, coronary bypasses, hysterectomies and prostatectomies, occur throughout the industrial world whether a profit motive exists or not. Drugs without merit, and many more that have no merit beyond those already available, are developed at enormous expense, which is passed on to patients. And doctors who devote themselves to the simplest, most effective measures of primary care and prevention are looked down upon by their colleagues and by medical students as non-scientific second-class citizens. In fact, they – not the overpaid super-specialists – are the true heroes of modern medicine, and we as patients and citizens should do all we can to see that they feel rewarded and encouraged.

Each of us has a personal responsibility not only to do that, but to see to our own care, to the monitoring of our own symptoms and illnesses. The saying that every person is a patient who doesn't yet know it is not just a joke among doctors, but a simple truth. There is no life without illness, no day without healing. What we can do best is what doctors and medicine cannot do for us at all: develop an active sense of the balance of health and illness within ourselves, and develop tactics for tilting that balance more and more against illness. Perhaps then we will be able to recognize that doctors are neither gods nor demons but human beings like ourselves, doing the best they can to help in any way they know how. A society that takes its own responsibilities seriously, that sympathizes with and respects its medical practitioners, is likely to find doctors who do the same in return.

C O D E
of S I L E N C E

Between doctor and patient there has always been a certain amount of mystery. Among hunting and gathering people, such as the ones I lived with in Africa's Kalahari Desert, the shaman or traditional healer offers little more than mystery, expressed in a kind of pageantry of dance and trance – and comfort. All he and his fellow-healers can do is dance for hours in a hypnotic ritual until the trance is effected, when they will lay hands on the sick, tremble and moan, and finally shriek piercingly as, according to the belief, the spiritual arrows causing the illness are driven out of the sick person, through the body of the trance-dancer, and back to the spirit world where they belong.

It is all they can do, yet it proves to be a lot, psychologically, convincing the patient that serious powers are being mobilized in healing, that weighty effort is being undertaken, risks are being run. In Western countries today we like to think we have ruled out mystery. But in fact as we approach the dazzling technology of the modern hospital and read of the wizardry of modern doctor-scientists – with their lasers, computer-produced images and gene control – we too are in the firm grip of mysterious forces. Of course, we say, smiling, but unlike the shamans of the past, *our* magic is real. Which would be a fine reply were it not that the vast majority of us, including doctors, routinely overestimate the power of the technology, and that – as has been endlessly proved by placebo effects – mysterious psychological forces alone often heal.

Studies have shown that the patient's state of mind affects the course of serious physical illnesses. Psychological interventions, including counselling and psychotherapy, have been shown to reduce recovery time from heart attack and surgery, and to lessen the suffering of patients in radiation treatment for cancer. Even a pleasant view through a window, as opposed to a view on to a blank wall, leads to decreased use of pain medication in hospital following surgery. In spite of the reduction in mystery that science has brought to medical practice, and in spite too of the numinous aura surrounding today's medical high technology, there remains a vital element of belief on the part of both patient and doctor that can have a powerful influence on the outcome of an illness.

The Hippocratic tradition of Ancient Greece was much closer than we are to the earlier beliefs in priest-doctors, so it is not surprising that Greek physicians cultivated mystery. Consider this passage from 'Decorum', an essay attributed to Hippocrates, who practised and taught medicine on the Aegean island of Kos in the fifth century BC: 'In fact, though physicians take many things in hand, many diseases are also overcome for them spontaneously... The gods are the real physicians, though people do not think so.'

There were also specific recommendations, apparently with a view to making the physician seem even more god-like:

> On entering bear in mind your manner of sitting, reserve, arrangement of dress, decisive utterance, brevity of speech, composure, bedside manners, care, replies to objections, calm self-control to meet the troubles that occur ...
>
> Perform all this calmly and adroitly, concealing most things from the patient while you are attending to him. Give necessary orders with cheerfulness and serenity, turning his attention away from what is being done to him; sometimes reprove sharply and emphatically, and sometimes comfort with solicitude and attention, revealing nothing of the patient's future or present condition. For many patients through this cause have taken a turn for the worse, I mean by the declaration I have mentioned of what is present, or by a forecast of what is to come.

The essay goes on to advise bluntly, 'Never put a layman in charge of anything,' and concludes that 'the physician must mark off the parts about which I have spoken ... For things that are glorious are closely guarded among all men.'

It seems an odd addendum to the Hippocratic oath: keep medical mysteries mysterious. Although there is clearly a motive of secrecy for the sake of the guild and its practitioners, the concern for the patient's welfare seems genuine in the warning not to reveal very bad news, 'for many patients through this cause have taken a turn for the worse'. In the United States today, a doctor who followed this advice would be on legally shaky ground. Until 1957, when the doctrine of informed consent was introduced, most American physicians still practised Hippocratic decorum; but after that date the patient had to be included in every decision with full knowledge of the facts, which in effect made the patient part of his or her own health care team. Over the past few decades truth-telling has consequently become routine, however bad – and potentially unsettling – the news, and this approach is being increasingly adopted in Britain and other countries, where doctors are legally free to use their discretion about what they tell patients but have responded to demands for patients' right to know.

Yet in treating patients doctors and nurses perform at least some rituals as much for the sake of the mystery as for any compelling medical reason. As for patients, they sometimes tell the doctor plainly that they do not want to know bad news, or at least that they are sure they will beat the odds. At such a juncture a certain diffidence in the doctor is advisable, however modern he or she may be, however convinced of the bad outcome. One of my teachers in medical school had been a Jesuit priest before he became a doctor. 'It is not the job of the physician,' he used to say wisely, 'to take away the patient's hope.'

One of the most impressive experiences in anthropology is to go to the other side of the world in search of the exotic and to find there a mirror reflecting your own society. Just as in Europe the ill among those of Christian faith have always travelled to holy places like Lourdes in search of spiritual and physical healing, so have many Japanese over the centuries flocked to Buddhist temples to feel the sacred breeze created by prayer scrolls fanned by the temple priests. Like the waters of Lourdes, this gentle breeze is said to be healing. And although it is very unlikely that Japanese physicians of the past followed Hippocrates, they preserve in their own tradition a strict code of silence that fulfils to an extreme degree the secrecy commandment of 'Decorum'. Most, and until recently all, practitioners have systematically and quite proudly lied to their patients rather than tell them the worst.

Take a commonplace example: Doctor Suda, a surgeon at a leading hospital, the Saitama Cancer Centre just north of Tokyo, has only a few minutes to meet with each patient. We come upon him as he demonstrates the lesion he has found to an older patient and her husband, shortly after she has undergone tests. The X-ray study of her stomach shows an ulcer, he says, and he points to it; she will need an operation to make her better. It is difficult to imagine the patient saying no to such an authoritatively presented piece of advice. Then the surgeon asks the woman to leave the consulting room so that he can talk to her husband. As the door closes behind her, he tells her husband the truth. His wife has a serious cancer; the surgery will not cure her, only prolong her life a little.

This is not sexism – had the cancer been the husband's, his wife would have been told the truth, while he would have been left to guess at the facts or believe the story. Nor is it some simple guild rule, with doctors shutting patients out purely to elevate their own importance. Rather, it is an ostensibly noble collusion among doctors, patients and family members to shield the one who is sick from the harshest truths. As medical anthropologist Margaret Lock points out, it would be quite unacceptable in Japan to tell the patient the truth, since the truth could be considered an assault intended to cause harm. The Japanese, Lock notes, 'believe very strongly that one has to try and bolster the feelings of the patient up to the very last minute':

> If the patient is psychologically strong, if they keep their mental state in good shape, then there is a chance that they can overcome the illness for much longer. There's a word in Japanese, which is *ganbatte* – the patient must work hard to try and overcome it. The Japanese feel quite strongly that if they actually tell the patient that they've got cancer, this is going to reduce their ability to fight the illness. Because in the minds of most people, cancer is a death sentence.

A similar attitude often holds in other cultures, if not in such extreme form. But in Japan utter insistence on the hope of a good outcome is a tradition arising from Buddhist religious belief; an optimistic mood may make the difference between life and death. Whispers behind the patient's back, far from being treacherous, are instances of tender concern. The truth will make itself plain soon enough; meanwhile all who really care will help nurture hope, since hopelessness, all agree, would clearly shorten life.

But the drawbacks of this approach soon become evident. Patients will not really be convinced. Friends and relatives have been told tales before, and have shortly died from their 'ulcers' and other 'minor' conditions. Some patients welcome the lie, some resent it, some even laugh at it – like Mrs Fusako Otani, an irrepressible, charming woman at the Saitama centre who chatted to all who would listen about the likelihood that she had a fatal cancer. Soon she was seen by the staff as undermining the lies they had been telling all the other patients, and the physicians and nursing staff called a meeting specifically to regain control of the situation, for the woman was challenging their structure of falsehood. Indeed, in addition to the usual meetings of health care professionals to review the treatment of individual cases, the (hospital) staff routinely review together the lies they have told to different patients, in order to maintain a consistent pretence.

In the eyes of many Westerners, such blanket withholding of the truth looks outrageous. What could be more threatening to a person's rights than not knowing things at once so personal and momentous? Yet until very recently Western physicians concealed the facts from patients as long as they could, often whispering the truth to the next of kin. Indeed in some countries, like Spain, they still conceal it, and in Britain doctors still frequently use euphemisms to veil or soften a harsh diagnosis. Gradually, however, because of an increasing recognition of the patient's right to know, British doctors have begun to reveal the truth to the patient, while American physicians, aware of the threat of legal action if they do not do so, have found it more and more necessary to disclose all the details. Simultaneously, doctors have increasingly doubted the value of mystery. Science has become the key to health and illness; patients can theoretically master some of this science and then take responsibility for helping the doctor fight or manage the illness. The doctor has to be in part a teacher of human biology, there to dispel mystery, not cultivate it.

At least in theory. In reality mystery remains, but it has a different location: it lives on the frontier of technology. Computed tomography, magnetic resonance imaging, laser surgery, laparoscopy, television-assisted microsurgery, lithotripsy, radioactive isotope tracing, radiotherapy – these are only a few of the state-of-the-art methods that doctors love and patients increasingly demand. These methods often work, but they are very expensive, and they are certainly not always cost-effective. However, they do virtually guarantee mystery; in fact the way they work is usually beyond the technological grasp of the doctors who make use of them. Only some engineers and physicists understand them. Doctor and patient stand together, grateful and humbled, before what seem to be technological gods; we are all awed by the overriding enigma of the Machine.

Medical systems around the world differ greatly, but all modern ones have this in common: a relentless pressure to adopt new technology. Although the Japanese have their code of silence, their patient-processing assembly lines and their struggle with health care costs, they also have their counterpart of the old-fashioned country doctor. Doctor Taizan Mikawa, a recently retired general practitioner in the mountain town of Nasu, is the eighteenth physician in his family lineage. His eldest son is a doctor, and his father was as well. 'My father was a real country doctor, and he was a wonderful doctor... He must have had some gift, not something to do with science, but something to do with trust.' Doctor Mikawa has tried to follow in his father's footsteps, and he would love to see his son follow in his; but fulfilment of this last wish may not be possible, as Japan moves into increasing specialization and hospital-based technology.

Another lifelong rural practitioner is Doctor Hideo Ozawa, who has spent forty years among rice planters in a mountain district. He is an old man now, but he has practised in this village since he was fresh out of medical training. He is the sole doctor here, and all of the townspeople, at least theoretically, are his patients. Some who could now be considered older adults were born into his hands, and he has tended five generations in some families. He knows his patients and their relatives as friends, has ceased to charge fees to some of them, and knows the context and meaning of virtually every illness. His dedication exemplifies the statement of his fellow rural practitioner Doctor Mikawa: 'When an old person dies, you cry with their family.'

And he makes house calls, lots of them – something now almost unknown in the States, though not in Britain, where GPs serving the local community are still the basis of the health care system. He even gives advice to patients he passes on the street. But increasingly the patients he visits are only the old, beset by chronic illnesses that are slowly becoming terminal. He follows them, examines them, chats with them and their families, gives what corrective medicines he can and, certainly, palliates their pain. They seem glad to have his care while they are dying.

It is not that there are no young people in the town, nor even that the young suspect his admittedly ageing skills. Rather, like people throughout the industrial world, they are dazzled by medical technology. They get in their cars and drive for hours to a big-city hospital, such as the Saitama Cancer Centre, which sees many patients with suspected cancer (in addition to the ones who *think* they don't have cancer). There they sit or stand in crowded waiting rooms, always for hours, sometimes for an entire day, until they can spend three to five minutes with a doctor they have never seen and may never see again. Why? Because they believe in the big-city hospitals, in the famous-name medical centres, and perhaps above all, in the magic of the technology. Yet the Japanese report the lowest levels of satisfaction with their doctors of any industrial nation in the world.

The Japanese are not unique, of course. On the contrary, they exemplify problems that affect medical care in all modern countries: confusion about how much money to spend, and about where to put the emphasis; excessive faith in science and technology – some faith is certainly justified, but ours is still excessive; and a decreasing emphasis on the traditional – or indeed *any* – doctor-patient relationship. We are a long way from that Kalahari ritual of healing, in which the earthly passion and transcendental risk of the healer creates a 'doctor'-patient relationship that in itself is thought to be healing. Yet some voices are being raised in Western countries on behalf of a revival of such a relationship.

One of these is that of Doctor Bernie Siegel, a former surgeon in the clinical faculty of the Yale University School of Medicine. After treating countless cancer patients with the knife, he became convinced that the patients themselves had an even more important instrument: the will to live. Looking back over his surgical career, he thought he could see a pattern in which patients who gave up on their own powers and placed their future entirely in the doctor's hands frequently died, and others who seemed to take their destiny in their own hands frequently lived. Siegel changed careers and became an inspirational writer and speaker, dedicated to rousing patients' self-interest on their own behalf, encouraging them to challenge their doctors and fight for their lives. To emphasize his change of direction, he even shaved his head. A dramatic presence, he fills auditoriums with seriously ill people, and very obviously he inspires them.

Few medical scientists take what Siegel says at face value. Among his critics are Doctor Leon Eisenberg, a distinguished Professor of Psychiatry and Social Medicine at Harvard Medical School, and Doctor Sherwin Nuland, a respected Professor of Surgery and former colleague of Siegel's at Yale. They and others point out that there is little scientific evidence to support Siegel's specific convictions. All agree that patients must play a role in their own healing – taking their medicine on schedule, returning to the doctor for follow-up visits, changing their diet and other habits as recommended. But this is a far cry from the sort of mind-over-illness message that Siegel preaches. No one doubts that there is some important relationship between mind and body; animal experiments prove that there is. But what is it? What frame of mind should you be in to fight your cancer? Should you be angry or calmly accepting? Should you fully express your emotions of grief and fear or find a serene path through meditation and faith? Should you seek support widely or stand on your own two feet? No one, including Doctor Siegel, knows. Certainly, any advice we may be able to give in the future is likely to be much more complex than Siegel's simple exhortations.

And there is a dark side to his counsel. When I criticized Siegel in an American national magazine, I received many letters. One was from a woman who had consulted Siegel personally while fighting her cancer; she believed he had helped her and was very angry at me. But most of the others thanked me for lifting a burden of guilt from their shoulders. Either they or a loved one had fought cancer, sometimes unsuccessfully, and the main feeling they had got from Siegel was that they were to blame for the illness. One woman had felt after reading Siegel's best-selling book, *Love, Medicine, and Miracles*, that her brother's death was partly her fault – perhaps she had not loved him enough. Others felt that they were somehow responsible for their own cancers. This was not surprising; one of the questions urged on cancer patients in Siegel's book is 'Why did you need this illness?' I'm not sure what Siegel means by love, but I would not want anyone *I* love to face such a scientifically meaningless and potentially hurtful question while in the midst of a serious illness.

What about the stories of miracle cures, whether through meditation, 'empowerment,' attitude, massage or faith healing? The late Norman Cousins, a distinguished writer and editor who took a leading role among the new psychological healers, believed he had cured his own potentially fatal illness with laughter and vitamins. In his very popular book, *Anatomy of an Illness*, he described his fight with a severe collagen disease called ankylosing spondylitis, which affects many parts of the body. Feeling that the doctors were handling his case badly, he checked out of the hospital, stopped all his medicines, and put himself on a regimen of Marx Brothers movies and vitamin C. He improved, eventually recovered, and became a guru of psychological healing like Bernie Siegel, but with a somewhat less 'far out' approach. He got thousands of letters from doctors in response to his story, and even became a professor at the UCLA School of Medicine. For a decade until his death he was a supportive psychological advisor to seriously ill people. Over and over again in his experience he met patients who considered their relationships with their own doctors to be non-existent, cold or counterproductive. These people sought and accepted a relationship with Cousins that filled, for them, a very disturbing gap.

What really happened in Cousins' recovery will never be known, but there are possibilities other than his own explanation. First, his disease is rare and not an easy one to diagnose; he may well have had a different disease that was self-limiting. Second, the medication he had been taking in the hospital may have done most of its work before he turned his back on it. Although discouraged, he may actually have left the hospital in pretty good medical shape. Finally, many multi-system diseases have erratic courses; they come and go, worsen and improve, almost as if by whim.

And then there is his belief that laughter and vitamin C did the trick. This is not impossible. There is an enormous amount that doctors and scientists do not know about disease, and occasionally a sick person may try this and that and stumble on something that works. Aspirin, digitalis and some other important drugs originated in folk wisdom and only *later* were adopted by the medical profession – which proceeded to take full credit for these old home remedies. As for laughter, well … maybe. And maybe too for warmth, supportive relationships, stiff upper lips, prayer, crying it out, laying on hands, and anger. And perhaps decorum, the Hippocratic code of silence, can either help or hurt depending on the individual.

There have been hundreds of experiments with animals and studies of people showing that psychological factors – things in the mind – affect the body, including the immune system – the molecules and cells we mobilize to fight off illness. Unfortunately these experiments have not fallen into any pattern that is useful for guiding the doctor-patient relationship, or the kinds of mental states that help the body defend itself. We can say that there is such a relationship, but we don't know what it is or how it works. These experiments are however used by Siegel, Cousins and others to justify very specific recommendations for seriously ill people to follow.

Perhaps a fairer approach would be to say: almost every patient needs to believe that his or her doctor really cares, at least a little; that the doctor's effort is a serious one, mobilizing powerful resources on the patient's behalf; and that if the treatment fails, it will not be because the doctor omitted some reasonable approach that might have worked.

One does not have to go to Siegel's extreme to recognize that all of us, when we are ill, need a doctor who will address the substantial part of our pain that is not physical. Doctor Eric Cassell, a practising internist who also teaches at the Cornell University School of Medicine in New York, has for many years called his colleagues' and students' attention to such matters. In an article in 1982 in *The New England Journal of Medicine*, 'The Nature of Suffering and the Goals of Medicine', in his 1991 book, *The Nature of Suffering*, and in his other writing and lecturing, he has steadfastly resisted the tendency of the modern physician to treat all illness as mechanical breakdown. In his summary of the article he wrote,

Suffering is experienced by persons, not merely by bodies, and has its source in challenges that threaten the intactness of the person as a complex social and psychological entity. Suffering can include physical pain but is by no means limited to it. The relief of suffering and the cure of disease must be seen as twin obligations of a medical profession that is truly dedicated to the care of the sick. Physicians' failure to understand the nature of suffering can result in medical intervention that (though technically adequate) not only fails to relieve suffering but becomes a source of suffering itself.

One of Siegel's recommendations is 'get angry at your doctor'. He harangues his audiences to refuse to take the doctor's clinical aloofness, the doctor's eagerness to get on to the next patient, lying down. He urges people to come armed with questions, to pry out the facts, to refuse to tolerate bafflement, to force the doctor to break the code of silence. He tells them to learn as much as they can about their illnesses. Up to a point this is not only good but wonderful advice, and it has the potential to improve patient care in many medical systems throughout the world.

For example, Doctor Julian Tudor Hart, a former general practitioner and a leader of GPs in Wales, has proposed a new model of the doctor-patient bond, which he calls the 'patient-as-colleague' model. The image is one of doctor and patient standing side by side, as it were, perusing the same facts together, exchanging views, planning treatment and prevention – in a word, collaborating. It is a far cry from Hippocratic decorum, or from the late Victorian model of the wise physician sitting behind a mahogany desk, delivering pearls of medical wisdom down to the humble, ailing supplicant. Tudor Hart's model – which, unlike Siegel's, contains no psychological speculations – could certainly stand as a goal for the doctor-patient relationship of the future.

Doctors can write the prescriptions, but they cannot come to the house three times a day to watch the patient take the medicine. They can teach exercises that will protect the weak back or knee, but they cannot stand over the patient to make sure the exercises are done. They can sermonize to exhaustion about cigarettes, fatty foods and alcohol, but they cannot physically stay the hand that is reaching out for these dangerous things. This is an ancient conundrum, and the ancient solution was mystery. There was something so compelling about the power of the physician, something so frightening and yet empowering about the physician's orders, something so comforting yet awe-inspiring about the physician's perceived link to the supernatural, that little or no understanding was needed to ensure the patient's compliance. And, since the theories of illness were mostly wrong, patients would have gained little by struggling to understand them.

Today, with the ancient mystery badly eroded, and with some theories of illness that are factual enough to reward learning about them, patients can be brought in both as students of the illness and equals in the process of treatment or cure. The doctor's role becomes one of teacher as well as healer. But as Siegel, Cousins and Tudor Hart all agree, today's physicians are very poorly equipped to fill any of these roles – teacher, colleague or, in the broad sense, healer. They are not taught any of the skills involved, from sympathetic listening to speaking in everyday language, from calming patients' unnecessary fears to inspiring them to play a major role in their own recovery. Nor, given the demands to be cost-effective, are they likely to have time to exercise such skills should they have acquired them.

Among the results are patients' confusion, scepticism, non-compliance and anger. Siegel strongly encourages the scepticism and anger. One result is patients who almost never believe what the doctor says. For example, Pat Pillsbury, a woman who had been in a serious car accident, felt inspired by Siegel to demand more and more information from doctors, and developed her own theories of lingering symptoms. She angrily went to one doctor after another – twenty-eight in all – in what was an essentially pointless quest, for it was evident from her questions that she was really looking for confirmation of a speculative and very improbable theory of some of her symptoms. Patients like Pat, and the doctors whose medical advice is unheeded by them, are both left frustrated.

However, unfortunately for simplicity, sometimes patients *are* the best judges of their own illnesses. One breast cancer patient I knew was especially diligent about self-examination. She found a pea-sized lump in her chest some years after mastectomy. Her surgeon had trouble feeling it, but when he did he sampled it by drawing some of it into a needle. A pathologist pronounced the sample normal, and the surgeon told her to stop worrying. She did not stop worrying, and continued to pester the doctor ('Whatever it is, I want it out!') until he acceded to her demand. When the little lump was excised and sent to the pathologist whole, it was identified as a recurrence of her cancer; the timely removal and radiation treatment that followed probably saved her life – and the surgeon praised her persistence. But the patient never trusted him again.

The patient-as-colleague model, in which maximum communication is encouraged, has the greatest likelihood of fostering trust. In the absence of this kind of open relationship, patients respond in one of three ways. First, they look for another doctor, demand to see another consultant. Getting a second opinion or even a third may be reasonable, and under Britain's National Health system there are not the same possibilities for patients to over-use and even abuse medical resources as there are when the individual or insurance company pays, as in the USA. But such distrustful patients moving on to different doctors, requiring more tests, further use of equipment, burden an already over-stretched health care system.

As will be seen in later chapters, all industrial nations are progressing towards a greater and greater sense of communal health care. In Britain and Canada funds are shared nationally or provincially by the government. Even in the US, except for the extremely rich, everyone will be drawing on funds pooled by private insurers and governments to pay for their treatments, especially the more expensive ones. And where there are pooled funds, there is mutual responsibility for careful use. In most countries doctors realize that economizing is not only a financial but also a moral responsibility, and in the future one of the main goals of the doctor-patient collaboration will be to guide this economizing. In other words, some patients will have to be convinced that the next test, the next consultation, may not be really worthwhile. The more they know about medicine, and the more they trust the doctor, the less likely they are to insist on being given expensive, inappropriate care.

The second response patients make to failed communication with doctors is to pursue 'alternative medicine' – unorthodox methods of healing. These range from faith healing to nutritional fads, meditation to chiropractic, herbal remedies to therapeutic massage. A few of these methods have received scientific support for certain purposes; most methods as applied for most purposes have not. Yet recent studies have shown that there have been enormous increases in the number of people who resort to such methods, that they cut across national boundaries and socio-economic and educational levels, and that few mainstream doctors appreciate how widespread the use of such methods has become.

According to a 1988 study in northern New Jersey, seventy-three different alternative healing practices were used by well-educated patients, all of them being high school graduates and more than half college graduates. In another American study of 660 cancer patients, more than half were using alternative healing methods; of these, eight per cent had never had mainstream medical care for their illness and forty per cent had abandoned mainstream care some time after starting alternative healing.

In Britain in 1981 there were an estimated thirteen million visits to a total of 7500 alternative healers – a 'healer' pool almost a third the size of the pool of general practitioners. A 1986 report of the British Medical Association found that 116 different alternative medical treatments were used 'reasonably often' in Great Britain, and by 1988 the Royal Society of Medicine was recommending 'bridge building' between alternative and conventional medicine. In France the use of alternative healers has become so common that the government has established a foundation to study 'soft medicine' and five universities offer certificates in it. In the Netherlands an increasing public demand for alternative methods has led to seven per cent of the population visiting unorthodox healers yearly, with eighteen per cent having consulted one at least once. Demand for alternative medicine is also growing in Australia and New Zealand; the trend appears to have spread worldwide.

It is as if the advance of science and technology, crowding the humane and the sacred out of mainstream medicine, has forced people to look elsewhere for the kind of relationship with their doctors that they crave. Although they are frequently deluding themselves about the efficacy of alternative treatments, and although some of these methods are simply dangerous, a few can be of physical benefit in limited circumstances. Some mainstream doctors are learning to take a tolerant attitude towards their patients' efforts to find alternative methods of healing. As long as the unorthodox methods can be more or less smoothly combined with the orthodox ones, rather than interfering with or substituting for them, doctors might be open to the idea of patients getting all the help they can get, including psychological help, which is too often wrongly denigrated with the adjective 'merely'.

In fact, one of the main reasons people go to alternative healers is that unorthodox practitioners are often more effective in communicating with their patients than modern mainstream doctors are. In one study of chiropractors, for example, they were more effective in helping patients with low back pain than orthopaedists were. But this was not because of their particular manipulations or other procedures; rather, it was because they had more success in getting patients to do their back exercises. Why? Because they spent more time explaining the treatment to their patients, more time teaching the exercises, and more time establishing trust. If it is objected that the time of orthopaedic surgeons is too valuable for talk, consider the cost of back operations for the patients who do not stick to their exercises.

The third way patients dispose of their resentment and anger is by registering a claim of malpractice. In the States such claims have sky-rocketed in a single generation, far exceeding comparable legal actions in any other industrial society. As has been aptly said by Bob White Jr, an American attorney who works for a medical insurance company, 'We are, in a malpractice sense, the equivalent of Beirut' – an image of relentless and often pointless crossfire.

In Britain until recently it was very rare for patients to sue the medical profession but now such legal claims are on the increase. Since people in Britain know that in a mishap their medical expenses will be covered, they have not been quick to resent medical errors. Then, too, they know that doctors are not accumulating great wealth at the expense of either the patient or the state. Still, studies show that the minority of Britons describing themselves as 'very dissatisfied' with the NHS rose from seven per cent in 1983 to sixteen per cent in 1986 – more than doubling the pool of patients likely to sue. Increasing workloads for GPs and decreasing time for doctor-patient contact are likely not only to further dissatisfaction but actually to foster mistakes.

But although doctors do of course make mistakes, few, even in greedy America, are negligent. Many malpractice claims cite doctors for what are really expectable errors, things that happen not because the doctor was careless, or stupid, or greedy, but simply because the doctor was human.

In addition, there are what used to be called acts of God, bad outcomes that don't involve any sort of error, that could not have been prevented even if the doctor were perfect. Malformed newborn babies, to take an especially tragic example, are usually in this category. Yet many malpractice claims after such births have stretched the facts to try to blame some act or omission of the doctor for the tragedy. The result is that obstetricians have among the highest rates of mal-practice claims of any medical specialty in America, and they are consequently leaving obstetrics by the thousands.

White's advice to doctors often boils down to maintaining a caring doctor-patient relationship: 'the fact of the matter is, we don't sue people we like.' The United States is, however, the most litigious of modern nations in general, and its people are particularly aware of their right to go to the courts for satisfaction when things go wrong with their lives. And although the rich have more of the knowledge and social connections needed to sue, enterprising litigators who work for contingency fees are aggressively reaching out to poorer patients who may feel, or be, wronged by a doctor. Juries confronted with a disabled person who is claiming physician negligence empathize with the person's need for compensation, and they are not deterred by the sums demanded of the physician and the insurance company. The result is often a multimillion-dollar settlement, of which the lawyer gets up to half. But, ironically, studies have shown that only a small fraction of doctors' acts of negligence result in malpractice claims, and many of the actual claims, including the successful suits, do *not* involve negligence. Thus the system neither does justice to the injured nor effectively identifies negligent doctors, the size of some settlements notwithstanding.

Yet the fear of being sued dogs every single US doctor, and is beginning to shadow doctors in other countries. Since the quality of the medicine being practised does not correlate well with the chance of being sued, it follows that every American physician must anticipate a legal action. No stone can be left unturned in the effort to diagnose and treat the patient. Some of the stones cost a great deal of money to turn over and have very little likelihood of uncovering something new, but doctors turn them over anyway, with the patient's lawyer in mind. This is called defensive medicine, and it now accounts for a substantial minority of the tests and procedures done by US doctors.

Successful defence against a lawsuit is in any case always a pyrrhic victory for the doctor. The cost in time, effort, emotion, money and damage to morale is very great. Even if the fear of lawsuits never becomes a reality, it undermines the doctor-patient relationship by eroding the doctor's trust in the patient. And the publicity given to jury decisions and settlements adds to other patients' mistrust of their doctors. It is thus a strange irony that in the era in which medicine's effectiveness is greater than it has ever been, the mutual trust between doctors and patients has largely broken down.

Although this breakdown of trust is a relatively new phenomenon, and the code of silence an old one, there is an often unrecognized role played by medical training in the estrangement. For example, after intense study and competition to enter medical school, the very first practical experience students have is often in the anatomy laboratory. These fresh-faced acolytes, having attained stage one of their dream – and before holding a stethoscope, a reflex hammer, or a patient's hand – are sent into a room full of strong-smelling formaldehyde-soaked corpses. Of course, dissecting a cadaver is essential for doctors-in-training and has been considered essential for centuries.

But something deliberate and important is happening here besides learning the structure of the body; it is part of what has been called the 'latent curriculum'. Students and teachers alike know that this is a crucial step in the initiation process, a way of immediately separating even the youngest people in medicine from all who are on the outside. It is the first real *we-they* experience, the first event that makes medical students conscious that they are not like other people, and will never be again. The mood in the lab alternates between high seriousness and rather sick joking – understandable given the stress of an experience which none of the students is supposed to reveal is stressful.

From my own anatomy lab I recall the group of students who named their cadaver 'Shop', so that at the end of each long afternoon one of them could say, 'Well, it's time to close up Shop.' Other remarks ranged from 'Chopped liver, anyone?' to 'I don't think this guy's gonna be playing tennis this weekend.' Except for a solemn but cursory speech by one of the professors at the outset, no attention was given to the psychological side of this learning process. But clearly each and every one of us was learning more than anatomy. We were learning to feel comfortable slowly and carefully dismantling the bodies of dead people. We were learning to hold sophisticated scientific discussions while handling parts of those bodies and blinking away the sting of formaldehyde in our eyes. We were learning not to think of the bodies as people but as a more or less organized structure of organs and tissues.

In short, we were having our first lesson in keeping emotional distance. This patient would not nag us with questions, show fear or anger, or cry out and get teary-eyed when something really hurt. By some lights we were dealing with the very best patient we would ever have: no psychological complications, no back-talk and total cooperation with all the procedures we needed to carry out. In some sense, cadaver dissection became a model for future relationships with patients, in which we would try to keep our scientific wits about us, suppressing all emotion while 'dissecting' and solving the patient's physical problem as quickly as possible.

If we became emotionally capable of treating the patient as something like a dead, unknown person – an intricate structure going somehow wrong, a puzzling, endlessly fascinating, broken machine – then our minds could win the contest of diagnosis and treatment, win the fight against the disease, without interference from our feelings. Although there was apparently no cadaver dissection in Ancient Greece, our modern version of Hippocratic decorum, which one famous physician made almost a cult of equanimity, could be seen as a systematic attempt to manage away feelings, our own as well as the patient's. And there is a reminder of the group of first-year students gingerly encircling their cadaver in the spectacle of a circle of doctors standing around a critically ill patient with tubes in every orifice, unable to speak even if conscious, the target of all of modern science's magical, often effective, yet sometimes dehumanizing power.

The hospital-based training of the modern doctor, driven by the twin stresses of rapidly changing technology and enormous overwork, carries forward the emotional distancing of the young doctor from patients. What is already a we-they distinction in the anatomy lab becomes an us-versus-them confrontation in clinical training. It's not that student doctors start out thinking of patients as the enemy; rather, the process of clinical training with its extremes of sleep deprivation, mountains of paperwork, endless new science to learn and a patient load systematically made so excessive that Hippocrates himself might well lose his decorum, all this instils in the young doctor a sense that his or her own survival is at stake. Eventually, as they often put it themselves, the doctor has to go on 'automatic pilot', processing the patient through the stages of treatment as quickly and efficiently as possible. There is little time for courtesy and no time for considering feelings – on either side.

More important, there is on the part of the young doctor an essential, self-preserving anger, and much of this anger gets directed against patients. It is the patient who rouses you from your desperately needed sleep. It is the patient who is 'trying to die' in the emergency room despite your best efforts to postpone this finale. It is the patient who often does not appreciate your efforts. And it is the patient who so often goes out of the hospital to return to the habits that brought on the illness in the first place. Doctors change inside during training; increasing cynicism is documented. From the 1961 book by Howard Becker and his colleagues, *Boys in White: Student Culture in Medical School*, to Terri Mizrahi's 1986 study *Getting Rid of Patients: Contradictions in the Socialization of Physicians*, observers have described and measured the effects of what has been called the 'punishment theory' of medical training. As one young doctor told Mizrahi in the early 1980s, 'You start regarding patients as the enemy and you really don't care.' And as will be seen in the next chapter, the process was basically no different in 1991.

Although when doctors go into practice the patient load is usually manageable and the sleepless nights are probably few and far between, a transparent wall has been built between doctor and patients, a wall made of science, decorum and silence. Most doctors care about their patients, they really do their best for them, but patients are on the other side and that is where they usually stay.

Tudor Hart's patient-as-colleague model has been adopted by some American physicians as a response to the threat of malpractice suits.

The idea is that if you let the patient in on all the information you have, if you make the patient feel as if the two of you are making all the important decisions together – or even that you are turning these decisions over to the patient – then you can scarcely be asked to shoulder the blame yourself when things come out wrong. The patient's lawyer can still ask whether you let the patient know all the risks of the procedure, but you will have an answer: Yes. We discussed the risks and the alternatives in detail. In fact, you could even say, the patient, given all the relevant information, was the one who made the decision and chose the treatment.

Doctor John Wennberg of the Dartmouth Medical School, an authority on assessing the outcomes of different medical and surgical procedures, has made an interactive videodisc to help provide this information to patients facing the choice of prostate surgery. Called *Prostate Options*, it describes the experience of patients who have had surgery for prostate cancer, as well as of those who have chosen radiation and other options, including the option of not doing anything. Although it is quite technical, at least some patients appreciate it, and it gives the physician a sense of not being alone in the decision-making. A lot is at stake: surgery frequently causes impotence, and can cause incontinence and other serious side-effects; and since the differences in survival time are measured in months, the choices are not obvious.

One of the surgeons who uses the film, Doctor Ian Nisonson, not only insists that the patient see the video, but he also spends literally hours talking with him and, where relevant, his wife, clarifying the disease and the treatment choices. This is not just a matter of avoiding malpractice suits, though he is certainly wary of them; there is also the relief he gets from collaboration with the patient.

> I'm not certain sometimes in my own heart whether or not a treatment is better ... there are times when I'm stymied. It is not because I don't know the literature or understand the facts. It is because it is a toss up, a fifty-fifty toss up, and sometimes I welcome the patient's involvement in helping me make the decision. After all, it is the patient's body that is being helped, cured, or violated, depending on how you want to look at it, and therefore they have the absolute right to make a decision. And sometimes it's comforting after you explain all the pros and cons to have the patient and the family say, 'You know, doctor, I understand what you're saying and I realize that I have to make the decision, because it's me.'

Yet even videodiscs and hours of conversation cannot give a patient a medical education, and may lead to false confidence in very partial knowledge. Also, not every patient wants to delve into the details. Some patients are greatly discomfited by them, feeling that they cannot quite grasp what is going on. They may need a little of the old medical mystery, the sense that the doctor is in control and giving the best possible care. Doctor Nisonson also points out that without some trust in the doctor there is no placebo effect – the almost magical patient improvement that comes even with sugar-pills. But at the very least the patient must take the doctor's point of view occasionally, if only to avoid developing unrealistic expectations.

Few patients understand how many decisions are 'a toss up' and how bleak and forbidding the landscape of disease can look even, or perhaps particularly, to those who know more about it than anyone else in the world. Doctors, scientists and journalists have given us all, including themselves, such a hard sell about the advances in medicine that only the most sophisticated people now go to a physician without overestimating what that physician can do. One of the best antidotes for the loss of trust between doctor and patient would be for patients to appreciate the limits of medical knowledge.

Medicine might be thought of not as a sleek space-shuttle rocketed into the perfect clarity of the stratosphere, but as a small and rickety aircraft taking off from a backwoods airstrip. Imagine that not long after taking off you are flying in the clouds. There is equipment for instrument-flying, of course, but it is not as effective as it looks. You can learn to co-pilot, or you can sit back and let the doctor take the controls; but either way, for much of the time, you will not know where you are or where you are going.

Today in Japan there is a growing minority of physicians who want to break with the ancient code of silence, and to enter into the patient-as-colleague collaboration style of doctor-patient relationship that is becoming more common in the West. But the danger of abruptly going to the other extreme is already clear in some cases. Doctor Yasuhiro Higashi, a respected cancer surgeon, after removing the breast of a young patient with a malignancy, met with the patient's family in a seminar room. He had already been frank with the patient, and now he was planning to share the details with her husband, her two younger sisters and her aunt. He sat them round the table and proceeded to give a lecture in a style appropriate – and no doubt developed – for medical students and doctors-in-training. It is unlikely that the family could have understood much of what he said, or of the technical diagrams he drew on the blackboard.

Then, astonishingly, he did something else that he would have done with medical students: he opened a plastic container holding the breast he had just removed. Pushing it forward on the table, he continued lecturing while pointing to the breast, trying to explain the illness and treatment for the relatives of the young woman who had had to give it up. He did not seem to react to the tear being wiped away by one of the younger sisters, or the frightened look on her face. In Japan, a culture that tends to conceal emotions, this small degree of expressiveness said something powerful, but the surgeon did not respond.

Surely the collaboration among doctor, patient and relatives does not have to go this far; surely *some* degree of Hippocratic decorum is acceptable – appropriate to the modern age and compatible with truth-telling. Withholding information is not the only imaginable kind of failed communication between doctor and patient. There are also failures of physician sensitivity, failures of compassion.

But then, the code of silence never worked quite the way it was supposed to. Tennessee Williams' great play, *Cat on a Hot Tin Roof*, centres partly on Big Daddy, a Southern family patriarch who has been lied to about his cancer, back in the days before informed consent. Part of the action revolves around his growing suspicions about the benign diagnosis and his ultimate discovery that he is dying. His response is not to get worse, fold up and die faster, as the code predicts. On the contrary, it is first to excoriate those who have lied to him for their 'mendacity' – the word is thundered by Big Daddy at all and sundry – and later to go up on to the roof of his mansion and glory in the farm he has given his life to building: 'Twenty-eight thousand acres of th' richest land this side of the Valley Nile!' Big Daddy's doctor is in the play, a foolish, almost pitiful presence who disappears from the scene when the emotional going gets rough; he is a minor character dwarfed by the sheer human magnitude of his patient and by the unforgiving power of the illness. He can offer diagnoses or lies, but he quickly and clumsily bows out when it comes to any search for meaning.

In Japan too drama has flowed from the doctor's code of silence. The central character in Akiru Kurosawa's classic film, *Ikiru (To Live)*, is told he has only an ulcer, but he deduces that he must have stomach cancer, a common cause of death in Japan. As he confronts his grief and pain, he slowly begins to try to find the meaning of his life, as a middle-aged minor bureaucrat with an average, distant, unsympathetic family. After an unsuccessful expedition late one night to try wine, women and song as an answer, a single obsession slowly dawns on him: he is going to take over an abandoned, junk-filled plot in his neighbourhood and turn it into a playground. Sometimes doubled over with pain, he works his way through the local government bureaucracy, quietly browbeating one petty official after another – after a lifetime in the system, he understands bureaucracy – until his persistence pays off and the transformation occurs. After his funeral, fellow bureaucrats memorialize him, trying to find words to praise the dull life he led. But these comments are belied by a closing view of the hero, rocking back and forth on a swing in the darkness, smiling beatifically at the small, impressive achievement that gives meaning to his death – and that will go on giving it meaning.

So the code of silence underestimates people in at least two ways. First, it is based on the dubious assumption that harsh truths always worsen people's illnesses. Second, it fails to give them their own lives to live and their own ways of giving meaning to their dying. Yet the patient-as-colleague model has its own drawbacks if carried to an extreme. Most patients need neither fairy tales to protect them from the facts of their lives nor a medical education to put those facts into comprehensible theory. What they need is a fairly succinct but compassionate account of the truth from a doctor who is prepared to help them through the darkness, either towards health – a temporary condition at best – or towards death, and to show that, at least a little, their sadness is a shared one. It would seem easy enough to combine these abilities with the skills needed to manage patients' diseases. So why is it so difficult to find such doctors?

CHAPTER 2

TEMPLE
of SCIENCE

The Johns Hopkins University Hospitals, Baltimore, Maryland, make up one of the very best medical complexes in the United States, and so in the world, bringing the full spectrum and power of modern medicine to bear on the health crises of ordinary people. Unlike at many hospitals in the world today, no one who walks through its emergency room doors is turned away. However poor people are, some government agency will pay *something* for their care, and however little it is, Hopkins will accept it. Federal Medicaid payments may not wash at some hospitals, but here they will suffice.

Whoever enters in pain and confusion and fear is met on the other side by people in white coats who will help assuage the sufferers' pain and probably improve their long-term chances. As countless people have crossed the threshold of cathedrals or mosques or synagogues, desperately seeking a remedy for illness, so we in the modern world cross the threshold of a great and powerful hospital. It is our modern cathedral, embodying all the awe and mystery of modern science, all its force, real and imagined. And best of all, it often does what it is supposed to do: it works.

A two-storey-high statue of Jesus Christ towers over the supplicants in one old foyer of Hopkins, beckoning them with a kindly gaze and inviting, open arms. If his pose is meant to be symbolic of this hospital, it is surprisingly close to the truth. There is a thrill being in these halls, to see the bustle of white coats, the stethoscopes draped round necks, the confident, purposeful stride of some of the greatest adepts and acolytes of the healing, saving profession. Perhaps we have to step aside in a long, harshly lit hallway as a stretcher is rolled past surrounded by rushing white coats – a stretcher bearing a person like ourselves, desperate and afraid, even now receiving some life-giving fluid that drips from a plastic bag on a rickety metal pole. And we may well feel awe, because this is one of the places in our modern world where we experience faith; it is, in effect, our temple of science.

There are other great hospitals in other cities, but Hopkins has a special place even among them. Medical school admissions officers in certain other top medical centres sometimes express bafflement at the number of students they accept but who decide instead to go to Hopkins. The reason is simple: Hopkins has an added mystique – its unrivalled clinical tradition. Here William Osler (1848–1919), arguably the most illustrious physician in American history, not only plied his trade but also spread a gospel that his turn-of-the-century colleagues found compelling. Henceforth, he proclaimed, medicine would be wedded to science. Hospitals would house laboratories and yet also be laboratories, and science would never stray far from the patient's bedside.

Adapting European methods of teaching to educate the doctors-in-training at Hopkins, he emphasized rigorous observation and recording of data. Students, acting as 'clinical clerks', were assigned beds on the wards and were responsible for taking new patients' histories. With Osler in attendance, each case had to be reported before the class as the students sat or stood in a semicircle around the bed of the patient. Nowadays the semicircle is never seated – it moves too fast, alighting only briefly – but otherwise Osler would recognize the ritual. It can still make medical students tremble – and leave patients feeling like objects being discussed above their heads.

Though most identified with Hopkins, Osler was born in Canada and is also claimed by Britain, where from 1904 he occupied the Regius Chair of Medicine at Oxford, and in 1911 was made a baronet. So he influenced medical traditions, and especially medical teaching, in all three countries. Osler himself, who is more frequently quoted today than any other nineteenth-century physician, once wrote, 'I desire no other epitaph ... than the statement that I taught medical students *in the wards*, as I regard this as the most useful and important work I have been called upon to do' [emphasis added]. This is from a man who, among many other achievements, helped delineate the nature of coronary artery disease and wrote a textbook on medicine that still stands as a model.

Today, in Baltimore, as in Britain and Canada, medical students are taught and teach others according to the tradition that stems from

Osler. 'Live on the wards' is one of the most memorable of Osler's many aphorisms. Hence the term 'resident' applied to Johns Hopkins house officers and registrars, and the demand that they frequently stay in the hospital overnight. Osler's dictum was: immerse yourself in illness; live with it, smell it, breathe it, be jostled out of your nightly stupor thinking of nothing but illness. You must wrestle with it as Jacob in Genesis wrestled with the angel; only then will you be fit to spend the rest of your life eye to eye with it.

Hopkins house officers are among the smartest and best-educated medical students in the world. Each one has been to school and college for twenty years, consistently excelling, and after all that, each has been chosen from many other excellent students who would have wanted his or her place. For the last two of those years, the third and fourth years of medical school, they have already begun to live on the wards, and they have been selected for Hopkins because of their pragmatic skills as well as their academic excellence.

Supervising them are some of the world's leading physicians and scientists, now bringing the Osler tradition forward into the future. Most of these are specialists who have developed and mastered knowledge and techniques that in their field are unexcelled in the world. Victor McKusick, for example, is senior enough to have been taught by some doctors who studied with Osler. He is the world's most respected authority on human genetic diseases – his encyclopedic textbook is the bible of the field – and he is also a dedicated teacher of young physicians. Not a few come to Hopkins in order to stand with him at the bedside, and many others wish they could. Doctor McKusick espouses the medical ideal of *aequanimitas* – equanimity – the title of one of Osler's famous speeches. McKusick even designed a tie bearing the Latin word as a repeated motif; it is worn with pride today by many Hopkins physicians.

Aequanimitas means poise in the face of a crisis, grace under pressure. If you (to paraphrase Kipling) can keep your head while all about you are losing theirs and looking towards you, then you may well turn into a good doctor. If, because of personal trepidation, a headstrong nature, excessive emotionalism or inadequate knowledge, you cannot keep your head, your calm, then you will make a botch of all that must be smooth and precise and competent. And if that is the case, you cannot serve in the temple.

Today sceptical voices are being raised about *aequanimitas*. Some claim that this ideal encourages callousness, distancing doctors from their patients and rendering medical care impersonal. In an eloquent essay, 'Against *Aequanimitas*', Doctor Gerald Weissman, a senior Professor of Medicine at New York University School of Medicine, takes on medicine's greatest cultural icon. Osler, he points out, was an arrogant representative of the upper classes; he was contemptuously patronizing towards his patients and favourable to the Social Darwinist ideology of his era, and he actively prevented women from entering medicine. A woman 'without urgent domestic ties', he believed, 'is very apt to become a dangerous element unless her energies and emotions are diverted in a proper channel'. He told medical students in his most famous speech, '*Aequanimitas*', that 'imperturbability is a bodily endowment' that some of them would never attain. 'The first essential is to have your nerves well in hand. Even under the most serious circumstances, the physician or surgeon who ... shows in his face the slightest alteration, expressive anxiety or fear, has not his medullary centres under the highest control, and is liable to disaster at any moment.'

It seems to be an early twentieth-century version of Hippocratic decorum. Yet Doctor Weissman doubts that this advice will produce medical students who 'will become caring, compassionate, or humane'. 'If the goal ... is to lead to *aequanimitas* – to teach control over our "medullary centres" – I want no part of [it]. The passion of the physician may be the best part of what we have to offer our patients and society.' And this statement is from a man who has treated patients with all varieties of illness, and taught medical students how to do the same, for decades.

Doctor Julian Tudor Hart challenges the Osler legacy in Britain on somewhat different grounds. He respects the concept of doctors immersing themselves in illness on a twenty-four-hour cycle, but not Osler's ignoring of the social conditions that produced the illnesses he studied and laboured over. Osler, for Tudor Hart, was the serene scientist who deigned to step down from his social pedestal long enough to minister briefly to the poor sufferer, bringing the alleged power of science (actually very weak in his day) to aid the victim in a crucial moment. Even with today's scientific knowledge, Osler's approach is inadequate, for it ignores the sciences of epidemiology and preventive medicine. He was not as scientific as he thought; and unfortunately, although science is much more powerful today, Osler's habit of exaggerating its power has come down to us little changed.

Perhaps this exaggeration was where he got some of his famous *aequanimitas*. In any case one can see the same process operating among young hospital doctors today. But defenders of the process say that doctors-in-training will have time enough to learn humane medicine when they go out into practice. In the teaching hospital, the crucible that forms them, they must first and foremost learn how to apply the science of medicine. In a departure from Osler's preference, they study mainly under specialists, who focus the utmost scientific sophistication on specific organs and problems. This, medical educators believe, will best foster a scientific orientation in young doctors.

Most medical students agree, but in the reality of training they often feel overwhelmed. First- and second-year medical residents can be on call every third night. That means they serve a thirty-six-hour shift, sleep for a night, serve twelve, sleep, and serve thirty-six again. If they have not finished their work by the end of a shift, they stay and finish it. Somehow they must also fit in clinics where they see a long roster of outpatients – those not staying in the hospital – and attend lectures and seminars to further their formal knowledge of medical science and enable them to stay on a constantly moving frontier.

They rarely complain (*aequanimitas* again), but if a dour look should cross a house officer's face in the presence of a professor, the senior physician may smile and say, 'This is the army.' Indeed, Hopkins house officers call themselves the 'Osler Marines'. After countless days and nights without play – twenty years of school, the last eight at their own expense – followed by three to five years of the punishing house-officer schedule at a salary of less than $25 000 dollars, or £12 500, a year, it is not surprising that American doctors are driven into highly paid specialities. When in their last year of medical school, still paying $20 000 or so for the privilege of being there, and with residency still ahead, the doctors' college room-mates of comparable ability who went to business or law school are already earning a six-figure salary. By the time doctors are through with training, they have a sense of entitlement to large salaries, besides needing to pay off the cumulative loans. Few of those at Hopkins, however, seriously consider leaving; in the US in general the drop-out rate from medical training is extremely low – around one per cent a year.

In the UK, many young hospital doctors are put off by the long working hours, poor pay and difficult conditions – which are not very different from those of their counterparts at Hopkins. At the end of 1990 Britain's Department of Health agreed in principle that an average working week for junior hospital doctors should be seventy-two hours, and that 'in the short term' they should not work more than eighty-three hours a week in 'normal' circumstances. According to an article in the *Daily Telegraph*, they were accustomed to working an average of ninety hours a week, with some junior doctors on duty for 124 hours or more – producing a state of sleep deprivation that they themselves felt put patients at needless risk.

The proposed reduction in working hours, even to such a high level as seventy-two hours, was widely viewed as a radical change, but it was not clear how long it would take to implement it. Doctor Angela Thomas, head of the British Medical Association's hospital junior staff committee, said that some in authority 'have had to be dragged kicking and screaming', and hoped that the new goals would be reached within five years – by the beginning of 1996. Meanwhile, in the US, under the leadership of, among others, Doctor Bertram Bell of New York's Albert Einstein School of Medicine, similar efforts to reduce outrageous working hours and increase supervision by senior doctors have led to new laws, at least in New York State.

If we enter the temple in the middle of a typical night, through the emergency room door, we will find ourselves in the midst of what seems at first to be chaos: stretchers rolling in all directions, blue-suited policemen rushing past nurses and doctors in white, the clatter of instruments and drug carts, the rooms abuzz with arcane phrases like 'This one's got four-plus ethanol,' 'Get me a set of skull films,' 'Hang the D-five-W!' and instructions from 'Just breathe in through your mouth, dear, you're gonna do fine' to 'I want some lights on *now*!' An amazingly calm young man is being treated for a gunshot wound while chatting pleasantly with the doctors; piercing screams in the background prove to be coming from a woman giving birth – here in the wrong, but not the worst, place.

The scene may strike us as horrific enough to be hell, or at least purgatory, but there is one thing missing from that time-worn analogy: here, people are helped. Almost before we get our bearings the bullet is gone from the young man's body and wonderful fluids protect him from the risk of wound infection that formerly afflicted victims of violence. Before we have time to become accustomed to her screams, the woman labouring on the narrow, rickety stretcher has become the mother of a safely delivered baby. Questions about why the young man was shot and why the young woman gave birth so precipitately – an obstetrics term that evokes a vertiginous fall from a high place, a fall without any preparation – have no place in the spare, utilitarian talk of the white-coated soldiers in the emergency room. They remove the bullet; they deliver the baby.

Osler again: 'Shut out the future as tightly as the past ... Let the limit of your horizon be a twenty-four-hour cycle.' Young physicians under this kind of pressure must relentlessly set priorities. But Osler's advice was not merely for a situation in which there is no time to think beyond today. It was rather a philosophy of how to think about disease and treatment; shutting out the rest of time and space was necessary not just for efficiency but for clarity.

Outside the inner sanctum of the emergency department, in the equally harsh, spare waiting room, patients with less pressing illnesses sit for up to ten hours in order to get attention they cannot get anywhere else. These are the uninsured, some thirty-four million strong, or about fifteen per cent of the population in the United States. These people exist because of America's peculiar system of payment for health care. Health insurance is provided through employers, who purchase coverage for their employees from one of approximately 1500 different private insurance companies. However, employers are not required to purchase insurance, and millions of fully employed people towards the lower end of the social scale have no health care insurance, just as if they were unemployed. Theoretically, if they are poor enough (unemployed and without resources) they qualify for Medicaid, a government programme that pays their medical bills. However, in reality this programme pays very little of what would constitute good medicine, neglecting in particular preventive or intermediate treatments before things go seriously wrong.

The American government claims that Americans do not have and would not tolerate rationing, but in fact they have rationing now, and one of the ways it operates is by making the uninsured wait. They lose hour after hour of earnings at work, and time needed for their children and to run their lives. They may or may not complain, but they do go home sometimes without treatment. Doctor Kenneth Covinsky, an emergency room resident, says frankly: 'This is really acute medicine, and there's a lot of very ill patients that come down here, with illnesses that haven't been managed in the normal outpatient setting. A lot of the people here don't have access to doctors. They come here whenever things get totally out of control. But if they were seen regularly a lot of these things could be better controlled. They wouldn't appear nearly as dramatic and exciting, but patients would be a lot better off.'

He is talking about the walking wounded. There are elderly people and children, people with broken limbs and people doubled over with pains in their abdomens. Many wait and wait and wait until eventually they are cared for. Is the hospital right in thinking these people should feel grateful to it, or are its critics right in saying that this is just not good enough? This question will be taken up later, but for now our focus is that of the young doctors: on the most urgently ill.

Rapid stabilization in the emergency room is often just the beginning of their story, which takes us deep into the strange night-world of the hospital. A junior house officer, Doctor Alicia Fry, who is in the middle of a thirty-six-hour shift, comes down to meet a patient: the Reverend Lilbert Campbell, aged eighty-six. She will later learn that he is a retired janitor and only a part-time cleric, but she will continue to treat him as if he were the Episcopal Bishop of Baltimore. Doctor Fry is a pleasant, pretty, soft-spoken woman who looks like the recent medical school graduate she is, but functions as though she had weathered years of rough experience. The Reverend Campbell is a sweet, weak, but alert old man who quickly rebounds from his astonishment that this young woman can be a doctor and places himself wholeheartedly in her hands.

This is a safe bet. Gently and deftly she enters a dialogue with her patient, and then with his son and daughter-in-law. She touches people, not just metaphorically but actually, hands-on. She apologizes convincingly for things she has to do that cause discomfort. She draws people out; she listens; she conveys real concern. She keeps her sense of humour and she shares it with her patients. None of these humane and human gestures impairs her efficiency; they all enhance it.

She soon learns that the Reverend Campbell has been dizzy, has had a feeling of tightening in his chest, has been taking a drug to counteract high blood pressure and has passed blood in his stool. She is aware that he is an old man with many medical problems, but she does not take any of them for granted. She begins examining him in the emergency room, but soon takes him up in the lift – personally, with her own hands on the stretcher – to the bed where he will stay under her care. From that base he will be followed and studied, with a view to finding treatments that will make his life both more comfortable and longer – at the expense of the US government's Medicare programme for patients over age sixty-five. Yet she knows that he has not been properly cared for medically – the way a well-to-do man of his age might be – and there are narrow limits to what she can do at this late stage. Also, despite her gentle dedication, there are other limits, the ones on what she personally can do. She says resignedly;

As an intern, you're in the hospital all the time. You deal with acute problems. You're very scared at the beginning. You're scared to death, the first time you have to take responsibility for a patient's life. I don't think it's the ideal way to train. It's very tiring. It makes you a little bitter, I think. You start to look at patients not as patients, but as a 'long hit' or a 'short hit' – are they going to be a lot of work or are they not going to be a lot of work.

She laughs nervously at having talked to a stranger in this rough-and-ready resident slang. But she does not let the moment pass. 'I think the intensity of the programme fosters that attitude. It's hard to keep your perspective.'

Another intern, John Townes, is on call with a medical student, Sanjay Marwaha. They are beeped to come down to the emergency room to meet Isabel Humbles, a thirty-nine-year-old woman who looks fifty. She is rather overweight, with a swollen abdomen and face, lying on a stretcher, moaning in considerable pain. With the help of some other residents, Doctor Townes finds out that Ms Humbles has advanced cirrhosis of the liver, causing her abdomen to distend painfully. She is a chronic alcoholic and drug user, and had stopped taking her prescribed medicine three weeks ago, explaining, 'I wasn't at home and I didn't have it with me.' She has not seen a doctor in some time.

A sense of futility floods Doctor Townes's voice as he talks about his patient:

> This woman has liver disease, cirrhosis, basically from alcoholism. She has swelling in her abdomen which is compressing her lungs, and she's having trouble breathing. She's got intense abdominal pain, gastrointestinal bleeding, she's not urinating any more. Thankfully she still has a blood pressure ... but she is extremely ill.
>
> Her prognosis is extremely poor. She's got multiple problems, and I don't think she's going to live very long, but we can probably tune her up a little bit and get her out of the hospital. When patients come in very sick, late at night – for some reason they always come in late at night – they can be a lot of work. I might not get any sleep at all. Probably won't.

He smiles. He is resigned, professional, even cheerful. He is doing the best he, or anyone, can, but in this case the best is not much.

Clearly the modern hospital invests enormous resources in salvage – emergency or urgent intervention to try to help people who are at the end of a long path of neglect. This is more true for the US than for Britain, and more true for the poor than the well-to-do, but it is a common problem in every country and social class. Conversely, neither the hospital nor any other health institution invests very much in primary or secondary prevention – measures designed to prevent illness before it starts, or to prevent it from worsening by acting early in its progression. At the same time almost all medical training in countries across the world occurs in high-technology hospitals, guaranteeing that each new generation of doctors will set priorities similar to those of their predecessors. And completing the triangular structure of forces are the poor, who under the US health system cannot turn anywhere else except to the teaching hospital and its doctors-in-training for belated free treatment when their lives are on the line.

How did the system acquire this structure, and why is it so difficult to change? In his 1987 book *The Care of Strangers: The Rise of America's Hospital System*, Charles Rosenberg shows that 'hospitals have never been ideal places in which to receive care'. From medieval times until the late nineteenth century hospitals functioned more or less like almshouses. They were refuges for the poor, the homeless, the hungry and, incidentally, the ill. In 1690, for example, the Hôpital Général in Paris took in 6000 people – one per cent of the population of the city – who included young men who supposedly refused to work and young women considered in danger of debauchery. But a century later, after the French and American revolutions, hospitals in the US and Britain as well as on the continent began to be more focused on treatment and cure.

Nevertheless, few who were not very poor would go to one, and the sick among the middle and upper classes would be cared for by private doctors and family members at home. There was still not much that could be done for most patients other than offering comfort, some relief from pain and, for better or for worse, some prediction of the outcome. None of these could be done any better in a hospital than at home – unless of course you didn't have a home. Although sanitoriums for well-to-do people with tuberculosis were introduced in the 1850s, hospitals and poverty remained almost synonymous.

The next fifty years changed all that. In the middle of the century ether, the first effective anaesthesia for surgery, was discovered and spread rapidly. Before then patients could be given only alcohol to blunt the searing pain; procedures often had to be completed in minutes. With ether much more could be done, and surgeons wasted little time in expanding their horizons to take advantage of it. In the years that followed, another enormous advance took hold: the germ theory of disease. In a painting showing the first use of ether anaesthesia, the surgeons are gloveless and garbed in Victorian dress suits, as if for a bank board meeting. Only after the role of germs was proved did sterile technique become relevant. Then, near the turn of the century, the X-ray machine was introduced, giving doctors the awesome ability to look through the body in their search for the causes of illness. And at around the same time biochemistry was being born, with its potential for diagnosing disease through measurement of components of the blood. Hospitals were becoming, in important ways, scientific laboratories.

Now there were reasons to go to a hospital even if you were not poor. Few if any private physicians could afford to assemble all these services in their clinics. Nursing became a hospital-based profession and helped to establish the scientific basis of sterile technique. Since nurses, not doctors, determine the quality of day-to-day hospital care, this professionalization of nursing was a prerequisite for the rise of the modern hospital. Centralization became increasingly advantageous for doctors, nurses and patients, and American hospitals followed the European example through Osler and became recognized as the right place to learn medicine as well.

Even a generation before Osler's, ambitious young American doctors often went to Germany to study. Clarence Blake, a Harvard-educated physician who had served as one of the first house staff at Boston City Hospital before volunteering as a surgical assistant in the last year of the Civil War, wrote home in 1866 describing the Vienna General Hospital as 'a small town of 3200 inhabitants' with 9000 births a year, where 'living specimens' could be pushed and poked more or less at will, and then in the end dissected. 'A year here,' he concluded, 'is worth more than many years' of private practice at home.' Doctor Blake was planning to become a specialist, explaining that the pace of growth in clinical knowledge was too rapid to allow for competent general practice, so he would pursue the deep, narrow knowledge gained from concentrating on one field – in his case, ear surgery; thus the pressure to specialize, 1866.

The German-speaking countries pioneered not only 'specialism' but a rigorous scientific approach based on facts about a series of cases and ultimately even on autopsies; these were the gold standard, since they were the ultimate test of hypotheses about the causes of illness and death. Rudolph Virchow, the Polish-born German physician who in the mid to late nineteenth century founded the science of pathology, can be credited with a role comparable to that of his contemporary Louis Pasteur, the discoverer of the germ theory, in the establishment of scientific medicine. As has been seen, Virchow doubled as a public health advocate, but his great contribution to laboratory science was to show that each true disease is an inherent, autonomous process with an identifiable course and a provable and specific derangement that could be located microscopically in the cells of the body. This delineation of one disease after another created a climate of unprecedented excitement in medical science.

One result was that patients as well as doctors, other health care workers and governments increasingly saw the hospital as the most promising and safest place to care for the seriously ill and, later, as the best place to give birth. The number of hospital admissions in the United States rose from an estimated 146 500 in 1873 – when the population of the country was about 40 000 000 – to more than 29 000 000 in the late 1960s, when the population was about 200 000 000. That is, while the country grew five-fold, the use of hospitals rose almost two-hundred-fold. 'Specialism' grew so strong that Doctor Blake's 1866 scepticism of general practice had become an article of faith and the ever dwindling number of general practitioners were viewed by specialists with increasing contempt. Some specialists, including surgeons, anaesthetists, radiologists and clinical pathologists, became largely inseparable from hospitals.

Yet despite its successes, Rosenberg notes that 'by 1920 almost all those criticisms of the hospital so familiar to us in the past two decades were already being articulated'.

> Concerned observers ... pointed toward a growing coldness and impersonality; they deprecated an increasing concern with acute ailments and a parallel neglect of the aged, of chronic illness, of the convalescent, of the simply routine. They warned of a socially insensitive and economically dysfunctional obsession with inpatient at the expense of outpatient and community-oriented care ... Medicine had to be brought out of the hospital and into the community – insofar as possible into the home. But such views were not to prevail.

The effectiveness of specialized hospital medicine grew ever greater. George Rosen highlights a striking 1938 comparison, by physician Alphonse Dochez, of the previous thirty years:

> He contrasted the histories of two patients with similar types of heart disease; one was recorded in 1908, the other at the same hospital in 1938. The total written record of the first patient occupied two and a half pages, and the observations represented the combined efforts of two physicians – the attending and the house officer – and of one specialist, the pathologist-bacteriologist. The record of the second patient ... comprised twenty-nine pages and represented the combined observations of three visiting physicians, two residents, three house officers, ten specialists, and fourteen technicians.

Only the naive would suppose that the rise of such intensive efforts of diagnosis and care is not a good thing. Yet increasingly in our era, critics within and outside of medicine are citing evidence of a point of diminishing returns, of costs that are no longer matched to benefits. Although general practitioners have remained numerous and effective in Britain – thus proving that they need not become historical relics in modern medicine – there too the rise of specialties, and of hospital admissions, has been very great. To a large extent increasing specialization can be justified in terms very similar to those used by Blake in 1866 – you just can't become good enough at all the different things doctors do.

Although specialists dominate medical training in Britain, as elsewhere, British general practice has remained not only respectable but essential; the GP serving the local community is the basis on which the country's medical system rests. But in the United States there is a very uneven geographical and social distribution of doctors, with large sections of the population – not only in inner city areas like Harlem in New York but also in rural areas – without primary care doctors. It is as if American physicians were an army without infantry, only pilots, tank commanders and other commissioned officers. Measures have begun to be taken to rectify this situation, including the establishment of 'specialty' boards for primary care and even 'family practice' – an updated, better trained form of general practitioner. But such programmes are not popular among medical students. Unlike in Britain's up-to-now wiser system, the US offers far too many incentives to leave primary care for high-tech medical practice. So the problem of distribution of care is nowhere near resolution, and the situation of the ill poor remains very grave.

Interns like Doctor Fry and Doctor Townes, as well as more senior, slightly less harried residents, must somehow find time in their schedules for outpatient clinics, in which the walking ill poor come in by appointment to have their medical problems followed. In the British National Health system people attend hospital outpatient clinics after a referral by their GP for specialist treatment; the GP continues to provide the primary care and to coordinate the activities of the different specialists. Yet most patients who come to the outpatient clinics of Johns Hopkins and other US hospitals have no doctor and unquestionably need to see one. But when they have to compete for attention with patients like the Reverend Campbell and Isobel Humbles, they just don't compare in importance for a resident. The doctor's most likely response is: let me do my real work. Doctor Fry and Doctor Townes cannot reasonably be criticized for giving these clinics short shrift; the system they live and train in enforces such neglect.

And their teachers recognize it. Doctor Dan Sulmasy, a young physician who teaches residents, says:

> I think that sometimes we have too much of an emphasis on the very, very sick patient. It used to be said that the best way to learn medicine is to care for absolutely the most sick patients, the way we do in the inpatient unit. But I think that's simply not true. Learning to care for somebody with exfoliative dermatitis, where their skin's coming off in sheets, doesn't prepare anybody at all to know what to do when somebody comes in with eczema.

This means that doctors who have saved the life of a hospitalized patient with a near-fatal condition are still unprepared for the day-to-day medical care that must be delivered by any general practitioner. They know what to do if your skin is falling off, but not if you wander in some morning with a devilishly irritating rash. Only a small fraction of all patients who come to doctors end up in academic hospitals associated with medical schools, so during their training the residents seldom see the kinds of problems they will spend most of their lives dealing with.

Although in Britain medical students spend part of their training working in a GP practice, most of it is similarly hospital-based, dealing with problems they may never see again and where the specialist knowledge to be assimilated is ever increasing and more sophisticated. And since British doctors-in-training are much more likely to end up in primary care, as GPs, the lopsided nature of their early education is at least equally questionable.

Doctor Sulmasy cites another problem:

> I think that there is a lot of frustration for physicians in dealing with chronic illnesses that are frequently not going to be cured by what's being done. I'm reminded of the ancient aphorism about what the goals are for medicine: *to cure sometimes, to relieve often and to comfort always*. And I think those are still truly what the goals of medicine are and ought to be – although we've distorted them to the point where we think we can cure frequently, relieve a lot of the time and sort of comfort when we get around to it.

This rearrangement of the epigram sounds very familiar to anyone who has spent time in a hospital, on either end of the stethoscope. An even more senior Hopkins physician, Doctor John Stobo, who as Chief of the Department of Medicine has responsibility for supervising all the other physicians on the Osler wards, acknowledges that he is not really pleased with the training he is giving them. He says simply:

> The way we educate physicians is out of synch with the problems they have to face when they go into practice. Our education still lags behind the reality. A number of the problems that end up in the hospital – somewhere around a half – are preventable. That is, by the time the patient ends up on the inpatient service, they have a problem which, if appropriately addressed in the clinic or if appropriately addressed with preventive measures, could have been avoided.

Doctor Stobo also notes that recent changes in government reimbursement policy – much stricter Medicare rules for how long patients may stay in hospital – combined with certain medical advances, have eliminated many important diseases from hospital beds. At today's prices for hospital care, you just can't admit the routine pneumonia or moderately unstable diabetes patient as readily as you used to. Such patients are increasingly tested and evaluated as outpatients, in clinics where the patients come and go on the same day. This means that the resident who mainly trains on the inpatient wards will today have an even narrower range of experience than the residents of only a decade ago. 'So we made a decision three years ago to try and move more and more of our teaching from the inpatient service to the clinic. Overall our progress has been much slower than I had hoped.' Because of the dual role of the residents – not just to learn, but to bear the burden of care for the acutely ill poor – walk-in clinics just do not get much attention.

Under the circumstances Doctor Stobo is sympathetic to the house staff: 'Their response to the patient with substance abuse, in terms of their feeling helpless, frustrated and in some cases angry, is perfectly understandable, given the training in dealing with those patients. If the residency training programme at Johns Hopkins doesn't become actively involved in teaching prevention to its house staff, we will be abdicating our responsibility to our patients.' This outlook is part of a growing nationwide trend in medical education, and important conferences have been held to discuss ways of incorporating much greater experience of 'ambulatory' or 'outpatient' care into the training of medical students and residents. There are parallel trends in the teaching of nutrition and other aspects of prevention. Yet in most places, as at Hopkins, little headway has been made. And since Hopkins is one of the places that sets the standard for others, it is not providing ideal leadership.

Doctor Robert Heyssel, former President of the Johns Hopkins Hospitals, certainly sees the need for change:

> Basically we, and I think most hospitals in this country, have been focused far too much on acute medical care over the years. It perhaps has more excitement to it. It's where we started really, as a hospital taking care of mainly acutely ill patients. The world has moved on, and while there's still a lot of need for that, it's very clear that prevention, and handling chronic disease appropriately, is a far more cost-effective way to do things, and basically better for people.
>
> We skew the residents', and in fact the medical students' experience, badly now, much more so than we did twenty or thirty years ago when I was a resident, in that most of the simple and reasonably common acute illness does not get in the hospital any longer. Most of the diagnostic work is done as an outpatient, so the resident doesn't necessarily even participate in that, and what you have in hospitals like this is one or two groups of illnesses: either very complex illness requiring an enormous amount of resources to take care of – cardiac illness, cancer, and the like – or in the case of this community, a very large burden of disease that is caused by behaviour and social pathology in the community. Certainly you need some of the experience you get here, but you don't need, I don't think, in the case of internal medicine, three years focused on this, with just a little bit on ambulatory care.

Doctor Craig Basson, an earnest, dark-haired young man, is an intern at Hopkins. His middle-aged patient, Helen Supik, is a diagnostic puzzle, in addition to being a very sad case. Her daughter Carla, a nurse, seems discouraged: 'When I brought her here initially she was still coherent, but within two days she couldn't move her arms or legs, she couldn't see, and was mentally declining. She's had numerous tests done, and we've really not learned much about what's wrong.' Despite her nurse's training, Carla was not prepared for such a medical failure. 'The first week I felt like I was in a nightmare, that *this really isn't happening*, because how can somebody be healthy one day and literally paralysed, blind and confused two days later. The next thing they're talking about doing is a brain biopsy; but I don't think they're real hopeful about that.'

Doctor Basson is asked if what she is getting has been the proverbial 'million-dollar work-up':

> Well, she's had the more-than-million-dollar work-up at this point.

She's had multiple X-ray studies of her head, including standard X-rays, CAT scans, MRI scans. She's had multiple invasive procedures – she's had a few spinal taps, she's had a liver biopsy, she's had skin biopsies, as well as a whole host of other X-ray studies – CAT scans of her whole body really.

Some of her physical findings are quite remarkable, at a very basic level. Things like her rash are indicative of certain kinds of blood vessel diseases that are important to be able to identify, and for the students and the interns right away that's an important lesson to learn. But even some of her neurologic findings many of us were confused by, till some of the senior neurologists came by and explained to both the interns, the residents, the students and the attending, exactly what they meant. And so she's really been very educational for all of us.

Talking to his colleagues on morning rounds at the bedside, Doctor Basson is more blunt: 'We've gone around and around, and I don't think any of us have a clue as to what's going on with this lady. I think we're all in agreement that the brain biopsy is likely to be low yield anyway, but it's the only thing we've got left.' As Carla says, 'I don't know what they hope to gain by cutting open her head and taking a piece of her brain out ... I can't help but think that maybe it's fifty-fifty, that yes, they want to help her, and yes, they want, for their own benefit, to know what's going on – just for the intellectual aspect of it.'

To be fair, the consent form that Helen or Carla signed on admission to the hospital was in effect a deal about this medical approach. They could have gone to a non-teaching hospital, where little or nothing would have been done 'just for the intellectual aspect of it', but they hoped that the white-coated intellectuals at Hopkins would harness their curiosity and come up with something better than local doctors in a community hospital would. A community hospital would either have sent Carla's mother on to a place like Hopkins, or would have tried watching and waiting while stabilizing the patient to prevent needless deterioration. But for Doctor Basson and his fellow residents, learning is a major part of their job and their fascination with the rare puzzling case stems largely from understanding their future: they have their whole lives to see cases like Ms Humbles and the Reverend Campbell, but someone like Mrs Supik gives them a different kind of opportunity. She can expand their understanding of how the human body works and breaks down; with her, they can push forward the limits of what they, as doctors, are capable of doing. And even if the treatment is not necessarily always in the best interest of such patients, at least a few of their future patients can be grateful that they did.

Sanjay Marwaha, the medical student, presents Ms Humbles on morning work-rounds in much the same style originated by Osler. He states formally what everyone in the room knows: that draining some fluid from her abdomen will be a 'great palliative treatment, and she'll be relieved of a lot of pain'. He does not state something else that all in the room know: that this will only help for a while and that the relentless downhill course of her underlying illness will continue.

Doctor Paul Oursler, the senior resident, is no kin of the turn-of-the-century physician but he makes a statement worthy of the master at his best: 'Unfortunately,' he says, swallowing nervously – he knows that what he is going to say is not the party line – 'a lot of what we do here has to do with people who have had a problem with alcoholism, drug use, smoking . . . we spend huge resources in order to take care of the acute problem, and yet we're pulling those resources away from preventative measures which would really work.' He points out that twelve per cent of the GNP is being spent on problems which are not, in the end, medical problems. 'The underlying problem is poverty, leading to drug abuse, alcohol abuse, smoking, and lack of exercise and obesity, probably from poor diet. And I think all of those problems are going to be effectively addressed by people who are not doctors.'

Mrs Supik's biopsy yields no information, yet she begins to get better, for reasons none of her very numerous doctors can explain. Her sister, Lynn Simpson, expresses an understandable frustration: 'It's just so overwhelming that in this day and age, with all the technology that they have, something like this can happen and they don't know what it is. Every day I sit and think, I just cannot believe it; I just cannot believe it.' Carla, the nurse daughter, is more frankly disgusted: 'I'm glad she's getting better. But certainly, after all she's been through, you expect a little bit more – like for them to tell you why she's getting better, or how much better she's going to get, or what caused it.' Even Doctor Basson, in his first departure from his aggressive, enthusiastic stance, speaks of her case as 'humbling'.

Unfortunately, Carla and her aunt's expectations are naive. There is danger in the common opinion that doctors can now do everything and that illness holds no more mystery. It inevitably leads to a tendency to blame doctors for not having been able to, as it were, read God's mind, to understand and conquer every blow, every threat that illness offers, even death. As Doctor Sulmasy, the young attending physician, says with an impatient, charming smile, 'The function of medicine is not to relieve the human condition of the human condition. We can't do that! We're not about making people immortal.'

Sadly, the Reverend Campbell – seemingly stabilized and awaiting further tests – dies in the hospital of a massive, unpredicted heart attack. No one has done anything wrong; when he came in he was eighty-six, frail, beset by multiple illnesses, and for years not even in contact with a doctor. He knew that each day was a gift, and would probably not have been amazed to learn that his life was about to end. The sensitive and effective Doctor Alicia Fry does not in any sense blame herself – and she is right; but summarizing her experience as an intern, she thinks that she will probably return to the lab to do basic science research. She seems to feel frustrated by the wildness of the frontier of clinical knowledge, by what might be called the incompleteness of medicine. Her withdrawing from clinical work would seem a sad waste, but her problem is also common to many patients and their families. Carla, for example, despite being a nurse, cannot quite grasp how basically primitive medical science remains, and how much uncertainty there is even at best. It is often because of such exaggerated expectations that patients experience so much disappointment.

Isabel Humbles has the fluid drained from her abdomen, a quite painful procedure, but one that gives her immediate relief. Advised about the deadly threat of drugs and alcohol, she packs a bag, along with a get-well balloon, and leaves the hospital apparently improved; certainly, in much less pain. Yet no long-term stabilization is likely. As Doctor Townes says of her, 'You can't help somebody unless they want to be helped.' But no one in the medical world will try to persuade her to want to be helped. She will not get even the limited benefit of a drug rehabilitation programme, because there will be no openings in such programmes in her area for the next six months.

Only a few blocks from Johns Hopkins, the Reverend Melvin B. Tuggle, a traditional black preacher at the Garden of Prayer Baptist Church, may be saving more lives than almost any doctor in the temple. 'Is there a doctor in the house?' he intones from his pulpit, and the congregation responds in classic style – but not loudly enough for him. 'Y'all don't hear me,' he says. 'Is there a *doctor* in the house?' enunciating carefully and calling his flock to witness. Their voices rise again and the sound swells. Later he will go on to say that Jesus is the cure, but with a new twist on the age-old message. He preaches a God-helps-those-that-help-themselves sort of medical revivalism. 'Cigarettes!' sings this minister in a tobacco-growing state, 'they are an evil and we will give any one of you the strength and support you need to put them out of your life.'

Driving a visitor down what he calls 'the Hopkins corridor', the stretch of slums between his church and the hospital complex, he compares it convincingly to a third world country. It may sound like rhetoric, but his claim is statistically accurate, not only for the Hopkins corridor but for areas like it throughout the land. For example, Doctors Colin McCord and Harold Freeman, both of New York's Harlem Hospital, studied mortality in their hospital's neighbourhood, using records for 1979 and 1980. While mortality fell in the United States as a whole between 1960 and 1980 – even more for non-whites than for whites nationwide – it stayed the same or even rose slightly in Harlem. As McCord and Freeman stated baldly in their conclusion, 'Black men in Harlem were less likely to reach the age of sixty-five than men in Bangladesh.'

This was strong language, echoed by the Reverend Tuggle's claim that his similar Baltimore neighbourhood is comparable with third world countries. The Bangladesh comparison appeared in the *New England Journal of Medicine*, one of the most prestigious medical journals in the world. Physicians and scientists at the Centers for Disease Control were not surprised, since they have documented similar statistics for inner-city neighbourhoods around the United States. And the figures are worse than they seem at first. If you remove infant mortality and look at the life expectancy of a pre-school-age child, you find that life expectancies for both boys and girls are worse in Harlem than Bangladesh.

To attribute the difference to violence and drug abuse is less than half right. This was *before* the epidemics of AIDS and crack. More than half of the excess deaths were caused by the same diseases that claim lives in better neighbourhoods: above all, heart attack, stroke and cancer. According to World Bank statistics, the probability of death between ages fifteen and forty-five for black males nationally – slightly over thirty per cent – is higher than the same statistic for underdeveloped nations such as the Gambia, India and El Salvador.

Life and death in the 'Hopkins corridor' have almost certainly followed a pattern similar to that in Harlem, and today, *with* crack and AIDS, the statistics must be worse. The irony of such human desperation, such relentless physical suffering, existing right in the shadow of a great modern hospital, is not lost on the Reverend Tuggle. 'The closer you get to Johns Hopkins, as you'll notice, the more the health problems become viewable. You see people on the steps early in the morning with beer bottles, wine bottles. This is dope city.' The

Reverend Tuggle's empathy for these people is palpable, yet his is no message of dependent expectancy. He says after a pause, 'Hopkins needs to do more, and also the community needs to do more.'

Under his leadership, the community does. In the basement of his own church, volunteer doctors and other health workers come down from the temple to where they feel that they can do more than hold back a relentless tide of overwhelming illness and dying. And they do it free of charge. One parishioner of about sixty, wearing glasses, in a three-piece blue suit with a watch-chain draped across his vest, makes a steady progress from station to station in different corners of the basement: diabetes check, blood pressure, cholesterol. Now he banters with Lou Becker, a prominent Hopkins cardiologist: 'Do you drink?' 'Only when there's a good game on.' 'How about cigarettes?' 'No.' 'When's the last time you saw a doctor?' 'That would have to be ten years ago.' 'What do you like to eat?' 'I've eaten eggs every morning for thirty years.'

This man's cholesterol count is 315 (UK: 8.19), very high. Becker interprets this to him gently, and says, unfolding a pamphlet, 'I'd like to show you a few things about cholesterol.' Since the man's blood pressure is also high, he is given an appointment at a special hypertension clinic the following week. 'That makes two today, about the average,' Becker says afterwards. 'Walking time bombs waiting to go off. It's great when we can catch it before it happens.' If the man can get his cholesterol and blood pressure under control – whether with diet or drugs – he will postpone or perhaps avoid a heart attack or stroke, the sort of event on which Hopkins residents may spend hundreds of thousands of dollars without feeling that they have accomplished very much.

Becker, a high-powered researcher, was an unlikely prospect for this sort of preventive care. But one day his wife Diane, a Hopkins health expert who runs the programme with the Reverend Tuggle, took him along to a screening. He brought a scientific medical journal with him to kill time, but never had a chance to look at it. He was hooked. He feels that preventive screening has made him a better hospital doctor, and he now encourages all cardiology fellows – subspecialty trainees who have completed medical residencies – to serve in church screenings.

That such experience wasn't required of them in the first place is because the Osler tradition has come down as an almost entirely hospital-based pattern of training. The thinking for generations has been that doctors must train by caring for the extremely, acutely ill. But what this means in the modern teaching hospital is third-tier, or tertiary care, that is, case of patients who were referred by specialists to whom they had already been referred by primary care physicians – internists, paediatricians or general practitioners, for example. In this specialized, third level of care, patients have been passed on by doctors in the two other layers; those doctors either were not sure what was wrong with the patient or knew but could not do anything more about it. Frequently Hopkins physicians cannot do anything about it either, even after spending a small fortune on tests and procedures. Yet sometimes they can, and it is in this hope that patients have always crossed their threshold.

If they are rich, they usually get the close and personal attention of top specialists, as well as visits from their personal primary care doctor; if they are poor, they get the residents who are training under the specialists – supervised of course, but not as closely. And they usually have no one doctor corresponding to the British GP, responsible for coordinating the efforts of the specialists and for mediating between them and the patient. This crucial, comforting, sometimes life-saving effort is often lost entirely in the United States. As a patient said in an excellent teaching hospital where I was a medical student – she had already been cared for by at least a dozen specialists – 'I have no doctor here.' It is easy to see how a person can lose hope even when, in a technical sense, he or she is in the best of hands. This is all the more true if the system has taken no interest in the patient before the point when it may be too late.

The Reverend Tuggle's programme, which is called 'Heart, Body and Soul', attempts to reach those patients when they have more reason to hope. At his church desk he ceases to preach and becomes thoughtful.

> People have lost their faith in doctors. The old family doctor who maybe covered the whole neighbourhood, people trusted him or her. Now with high-tech 'modernology' . . . computers, etcetera coming into the hospital, people have become a number. It's machines that work on them, doctors do not work on them. The personal emphasis is gone now.
>
> We need hands-on, walk-the-street doctors, neighbourhood doctors. At one time we had a lot of practices in East Baltimore. It's gone now. . . . Doctors are scared.'

He also notes that doctors can't make enough money as general practitioners, so that most want to specialize. A bizarre system of payments has made it financially unrewarding to practise any but the most high-tech medical care. Private insurance companies have largely created this imbalance, but it has been reinforced by patient demand and by government; it exists to a lesser extent in Britain and other countries as well.

Physicians have traditionally justified specialization as a healthy trend that supplies the most expert care in the most specific way to the patient in the most dire need. In the postwar period, when many medical-specialty certification boards were just forming, this was true. Science was delivering on its turn-of-the-century promise, and miracle drugs like penicillin and streptomycin were controlling infectious scourges and making surgery unprecedentedly safe. X-ray techniques and other diagnostic technologies became steadily better.

But somewhere a point of diminishing returns was reached. More and more money was being spent for an ever smaller return, whether measured in terms of deaths prevented or of suffering relieved. Things were still improving steadily, but in smaller and smaller steps, and many people at length concluded that the price had simply become too high. Costs are, of course, always relative. But given a finite health care budget, whether too much is spent on hospital-based treatments that are expensive and often futile, relative to neighborhood-based primary care and prevention – the sort of thing going on in the basement of the Garden of Prayer Baptist Church – the answer is a simple yes.

In these discussions it is sometimes hard to be sure whether we are talking about the problem of acute, high-tech medicine, the problem of lopsided medical training, or the problem of inadequate health care for the poor. That is because these are inextricably entwined. Among doctors, only the young residents are on a low enough salary to be cost-effective in care for the poor. And because of their need, the poor will tolerate being the focus of training. Meanwhile, those entrusted with the training of medical residents feel very keenly the imperative of training those young people *on the frontier* – not just the one between health and illness, but the one between what we can do and what we cannot: the frontier of current medical science.

So does this mean, in the words of Mrs Supik's daughter after the biopsy, that half the reason these high-tech procedures are done is that they are useful in training? This is a great oversimplification, but there is some truth here. Everything that was done in Mrs Supik's costly work-up was done for her benefit in an honest attempt to find out what was wrong with her and open some avenue, or at least a path, of treatment. But while her intern, Doctor Basson, was being exposed to the remarkable array of state-of-the-art procedures invoked for her – exposure he was obviously enthusiastic about – he was *not* being exposed to primary care in an outpatient clinic, or to preventive care in the style of Reverend Tuggle's Health Fair. As his teacher, Doctor Stobo, says, if we don't train young doctors in primary care and preventive medicine, we abdicate our responsibility to patients. Doctor Heyssel, the hospital's former President, agrees.

These comments reminded me of the time when, in my third year of medical school, I felt frustrated, as Doctor Fry and Doctor Townes do, by the parade of acutely ill patients with irreversible chronic diseases. Why, I wondered, is everything we do so heavily reliant on high technology? Why can't we reach these people earlier, when we might do some good? Imagine my surprise when I read, in an issue of *Time* magazine, of the opinion of the Dean of the Harvard Medical School that 'Medical education is not in optimum health'; of the Dean of the Johns Hopkins School of Medicine at the time, 1983, that 'We would like to reverse the trend toward early specialization and over-emphasis on science as preparation for medicine'; and of the Dean of the Columbia College of Physicians and Surgeons that medical students must learn 'how to deal with the patient, the patient's family, and his whole life, rather than "the third bed on the left with a coronary" '. Listening to Doctor Stobo and Doctor Heyssel gave me the same stunned feeling I had had then: if the people who run the system don't like it, why don't they change it?

There is a profound answer: they can't. No one at any place in the hierarchy, however high up, can wilfully counteract the forces that make it work – or fail to work – the way it does. These forces include the steady advance of science, the cultural traditions of medical training (*I did it, so you have to do it*), the nation's financial need to use trainees to care for the poor, the insurance companies' misplaced sense of responsibility – greater towards their stockholders than towards patients – the bizarre patterns of reimbursement insurers maintain, the consequent disproportionate income and influence of procedure-oriented specialties, colossal administrative waste, greed and fraud, and the enormous impact of soaring malpractice litigation on medical decision-making.

But perhaps a greater force than any of these is what I call the 'what if it's your mother' principle. It is the principle expressed in the most haunting question posed by hospital doctors when they hear their system criticized. What if Mrs Supik were your mother? Would you want to hear arguments about how many lives could be saved through immunization using the $200 000 spent on her hospitalization? Or would you prefer that no expense be spared in the attempt to find out how to control and reverse this dreadful deterioration in a vigorous woman full of life and hope? What if Isabel Humbles were your mother? Would you want to be lectured about the need for her and others to stop drinking, and hear about the impossibility of getting her into a drug rehabilitation programme? Or would you want the doctor to stop preaching and just draw off the fluid that is choking her to death?

Every congressional representative and county official in the United States asks these same questions when considering how to allocate health care, and similar dilemmas over costs and resources face Britain's and other countries' health services. Most malpractice suits are driven by these questions, causing doctors to practise high-tech defensive medicine that costs a fortune. And the officials and lawyers attend to these questions because they are on the minds of the average man and woman on the street. Not, *Why is my child or* (even less) *someone else's child not immunized?* but *What will happen if my child has leukemia?;* not, *I wonder what my cholesterol level is,* but *What will happen when I have a heart attack?* Doctors are not immune to the compelling drama of the illness that has become a matter of life and death. That is why Doctor Townes feels good about himself, in spite of his frustration with Isabel Humbles' irreversible condition. Who would *not* feel good taking someone who entered hospital on a stretcher, swollen and screaming with pain, and who goes out a few days later on her own two feet? It is also why Doctor Basson conveys such enthusiasm for the next test, and the next, and the next – not just because he wants to play with the big toys and learn, but because he is hoping against hope that he and his teachers will find something that will make Mrs Supik whole and well again.

No one has a right to ask Doctor Townes or Doctor Basson to think about drug rehabilitation places or unimmunized children when they are standing over desperately ill people in pain. Indeed, at that moment such thoughts are irrelevant; as Osler advised, confine your thinking to a twenty-four-hour cycle, putting everything else out of your mind. But as long as there is a finite limit to health care expenditures someone must think those other thoughts. A choice has to be made about where to put the money; how to balance the columns of black and red ink. As dreadful and cold-hearted as it seems, we must weigh Ms Humbles' perhaps penultimate medical stabilization against the fate of other addicts who are not so sick but also cannot get into drug programmes. We must weigh some of Mrs Supik's CAT scans against the fate of the unimmunized children.

Recently I was talking with an extremely bright young doctor who was in the midst of a three-year residency – just like the one the Hopkins physicians are going through. She spoke with great enthusiasm about the same state-of-the-art three-dimensional imaging that excited Doctor Basson as it guided Mrs Supik's biopsy. But she also spoke with great enthusiasm about the satellite clinics set up by Atlanta's Grady Hospital to serve the poor of the city in their own neighbourhoods. I said, 'You cannot be equally enthusiastic about everything. Sooner or later we will come to a point where someone will say to you, "Should we buy another six-million dollar magnetic resonance imager, or should we build another satellite clinic? We can't do both." Which will you choose?' Articulate and experienced as she was, she did not have an answer – no indictment of her, since neither, at present, does anyone else.

CHAPTER 3

The MAGIC BULLET

At around the same time that William Osler in Baltimore was developing the American modern teaching hospital, Paul Ehrlich in Frankfurt was laying the foundations of what we now call chemotherapy – the specific treatment of diseases by deliberately crafted chemicals. His observations of diphtheria, a then-dreaded bacterial killer of children, had taught him that the body itself can produce chemical agents *specifically* to damage an invading microbe – a disease-causing germ – in a process now known as specific immunity. And his studies of lead poisoning had shown him that some chemicals brought into the body – in this case a toxic one – home in on certain organs. His hope was for new drugs that would go directly to a diseased organ or to a microbe, destroying the germ and defeating the disease with few other effects on the body.

He used the phrase 'silver bullet' to describe the dream chemical that would target a given disease. At the time he was working on syphilis, then a devastating chronic disease caused by bacteria called spirochetes. These he watched under his microscope while continually making and trying new compounds that might have a chance of specifically killing them. The six-hundred-and-sixth compound he tried worked dramatically, and was marketed in 1910 under the name Salvarsan. In the age of AIDS it is worth noting that Salvarsan, the forerunner of most twentieth-century drug treatments, came out of the search for a cure for a sexually transmitted, chronically degenerative, deadly disease.

Unfortunately Salvarsan was not quite the silver bullet after all, for it had major side-effects for those who were helped by it. On balance, however, the treatment with Salvarsan was undoubtedly a very beneficial advance; it marked the end of an era when many medicines were little more than generalized poisons, containing lead, mercury and arsenic. Yet there was equally little doubt that the search for a better treatment than Salvarsan should continue.

'Magic Bullet' is now our description for Ehrlich's concept, although in the strict sense there is no magic cure, for syphilis or any other disease. Every drug that has been of use against disease has imposed a cost on those who took it, in the form of unwanted effects on the body. Aspirin and paracetamol seem at first like magic bullets for fever, but aspirin may burn a hole in your stomach – or, if you are a child, may in rare cases give you the very dangerous Reyes' syndrome – while paracetamol may do permanent harm to your kidneys. Insulin seems at first a magic bullet for 'sugar' disease – diabetes. But by doing what it's supposed to do – reduce blood sugar levels – too well, it can produce a potentially deadly insulin shock. Penicillin is a magic bullet for, say, pneumonia – if you're not unlucky enough to be allergic to it. Even if you're not, it may still kill the normal bacteria in your gut, causing you indigestion; and more important, over time and many treatments in a community, it will relentlessly breed bacteria that are immune to its effects, taking you right back to the start of another search for a magic bullet.

In the end, what we are searching for is a self-contradiction: a chemical agent which acts powerfully on an illness – a living thing, whether microbe, tumour or failing organ – but which is completely without other, unwanted actions in the body. The trouble is that an agent that has powerful biological effects in one area has powerful biological effects in others. Evolution has not designed living things with absolute precision and specificity; it has been a clumsy process, utilizing random changes and building on what it has at any point in time – rather like a small child making a complex structure out of small, differently coloured lumps of clay: if another child comes along determined to pull out all the (say) green lumps, the structure will be vulnerable in many places, not just one. In the sense of absolute specificity, the magic bullet is a vain hope – the existence of effective drug treatments notwithstanding.

There is another, more important side-effect of dream drugs: they lull us, even in anticipation, into a false sense of safety. We enter an illusory world in which anything that is broken can be simply fixed, in which anything that is wrong with us has its own private molecular magic wand that, when waved over us, will make it go away.

We can smoke ourselves into lung cancer and heart attack, drink ourselves into liver disease, and eat ourselves into diabetes and stroke. We are fearless about these things because of a new version of the age-old denial of death. We inherit from our evolutionary past the basic animal feeling that says, *What is happening now will surely go on for ever*, and we add to that the ancient human tendency to ignore the future, especially if that future may be anything worse than the present. If a thought is painful, we decline to think it. But we compound these denials with an unrealistic vision of the power of modern science in the battle against disease and death. Deep down we think we have the system beaten; we will make it all right again at the other end of the story. After all, aren't we approaching the twenty-first century? Drug company scientists can do practically anything with those molecules and test-tubes, can't they?

Indeed there are millions of people for whom newly invented drugs *have* been virtual miracle cures. James Nelson is one of them. In the late 1980s he had begun to suffer from Cushing's Syndrome – an array of unsettling symptoms caused by an excess of the hormone cortisol, which in normal amounts is one of the body's main aids in coping with stress. This disorder can affect virtually any organ. One common feature is weight gain in the abdomen, the skin of which may develop stripes due to stretching. Bloating of the face, muscle weakness, fragile bones, thinning of the skin with a lot of bruising, lowered resistance to infection, high blood pressure, depression and impotence are all frequent components. In Mr Nelson's case, by his own testimony and that of his wife, his life had become practically unliveable, their marriage little more than shared anguish.

The syndrome is often caused by a tumour of the adrenal gland, a small, soft, pyramidal structure atop each kidney, which produces cortisol. The gland's normal function runs amok as a result of the tumour working overtime to make unneeded cortisol. This turned out to be what had happened to Mr Nelson, but the search for the tiny disease-producing lump went on for a full year. Only then could the tumour be removed by surgery, and this long wait would usually have meant a continuing and partly irreversible deterioration in Mr Nelson's condition; even if he had survived, his life would have been truly dreadful.

But Mr Nelson was lucky enough to have access to the National Institutes of Health in Maryland, where Doctor Lynnette Nieman and her colleagues were conducting a study of a promising new drug called mifepristone. This agent, they had reason to believe, would block the effects of the excess cortisol on a number of body systems, essentially

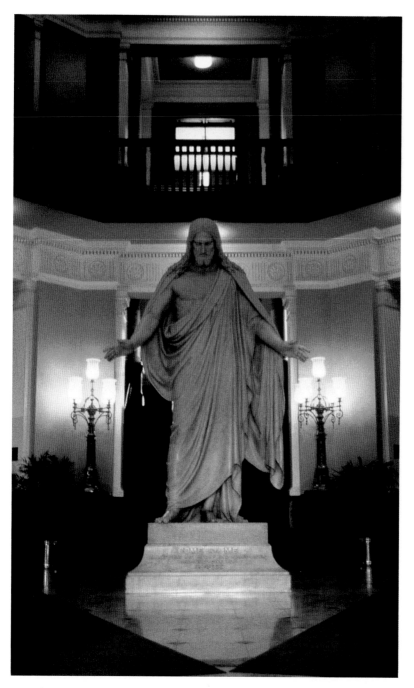

1 Johns Hopkins University Hospital, Baltimore, one of the world's great temples of medical science.

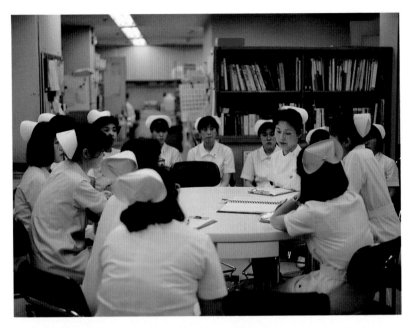

2   Japanese cancer ward nurses meet to discuss their patients: who can be told some of the truth and who should be told lies?

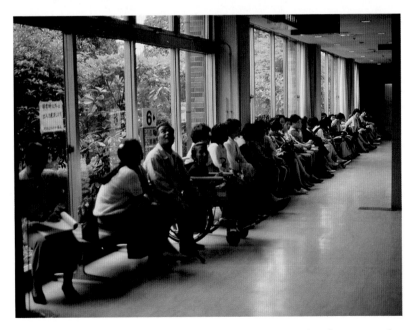

3   Japanese patients queue for hours, sometimes an entire day, to see the doctor who then spends less than five minutes with each of them.

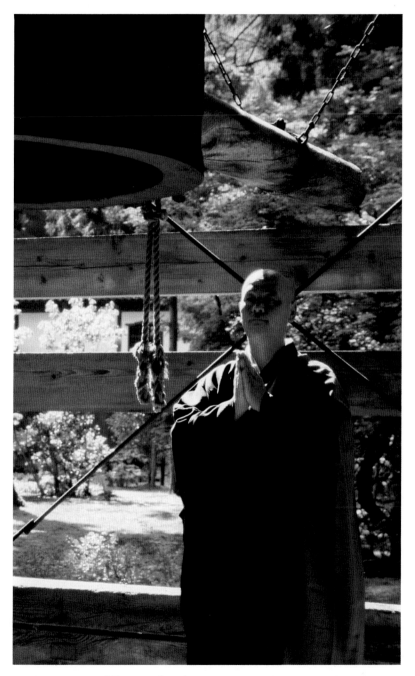

4   A Japanese Buddhist monk at the Untoan Temple, Nigata, calling patients
to a healing ceremony. For Buddhists, mind and body are inseparable, and
this philosophy affects all of Japanese medicine.

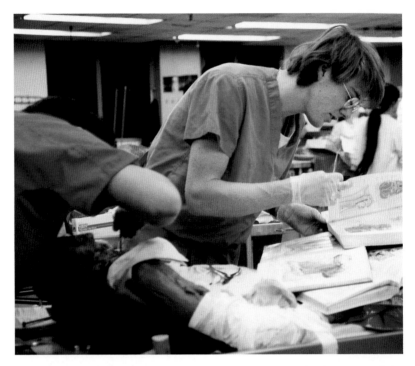

5 Medical students at Columbia University, New York; they meet their first patients – dead bodies – in the anatomy class, which often affects their attitude to patients for the rest of their lives.

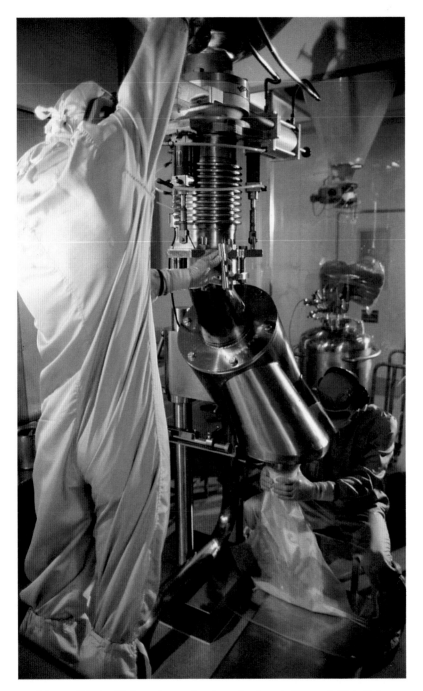

6   The antibiotic Claforan in production; the drug is Roussel–Uclaf's latest
weapon in the arms race against resistant microbes.

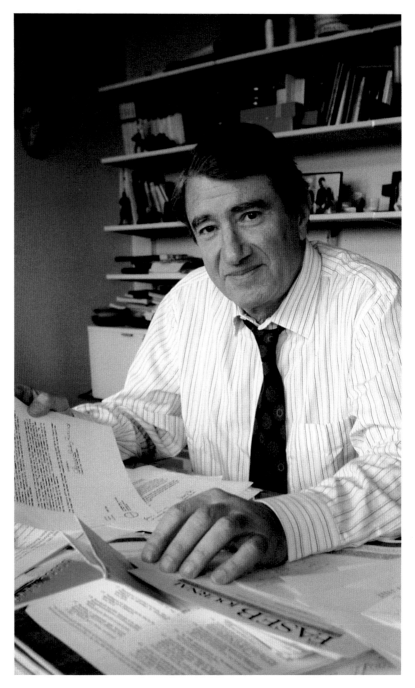

7   Professor Etienne-Emile Baulieu, physician-scientist, co-discoverer of the controversial abortion pill RU 486.

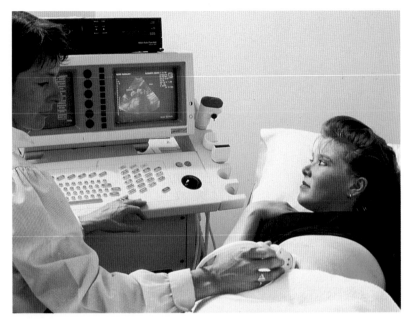

8 Hoping for a perfect baby, Elizabeth Hearne watches the ultrasound image of her unborn child.

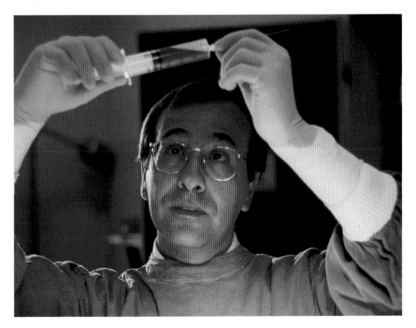

9 Dr Giovanni Monni looks at the results of prenatal testing for thalassemia in Sardinia. The incidence of this dread disease has been greatly reduced, but controversy continues.

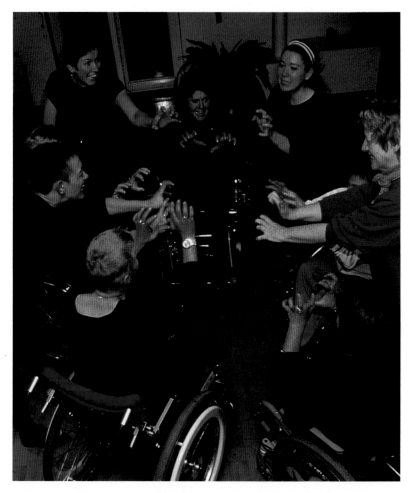

10　A self-defence class for disabled women in Bremen. The Nazis, using a crude form of the science of eugenics, sought to eliminate the disabled.

by tricking each organ into absorbing the harmless mifepristone while blocking out the dangerous cortisol. It turned out to be one of those happy situations in which a theory about the body's chemistry was in the event both correct and powerful. A molecule that had been dreamed up by a drug company scientist, at the blackboard and in the laboratory, was administered by a doctor thousands of miles away, and it reversed Mr Nelson's deterioration.

Since people with Cushing's Syndrome have lives that are unpredictable and short, it is quite possible that, as Mr Nelson believes, mifepristone made all the difference to his: 'I can honestly say that it played an important part in maybe even saving my life.' His wife is more definite: 'His life was a complete turnaround – it was like a miracle. To go from one side of life and then to see the other, it was actually beautiful.'

This kind of 'miracle cure' is not rare in modern medicine, but nor is it common. As was seen in the last chapter, most of the people who come into hospitals today do not have ailments that can be quickly cured by miraculous drugs. They have chronic, degenerative conditions that can often be slowed, or even stopped, by drugs, but are not easily reversed. And even when drugs do work, they carry a cost in side-effects that is often very high – sometimes unacceptably high. Have we reached a plateau after a century of uphill climbing? Has the advance in drug treatment, seemingly moving to greater and greater heights in every decade, finally reached a point at which future gains will be small? Will we continue to invent new drugs like mifepristone, or will our drugs of the future be more like AZT – another new agent, helpful to AIDS patients for a while, but only a while, and really only postponing the inevitable?

In a sense, ether was the first great modern drug; introduced in the 1840s, it caused a state of painless and safe unconsciousness that transformed the possiblities of surgical cure – functions that from ancient times were served by natural substances like alcohol and opium. But ether was an adjunct to treatment, not really a treatment itself. Quinine, a tree-bark product known to be useful in combating malaria, may have been the first commercially marketed drug treatment, but aspirin probably has the honour of being the first truly mass-produced drug. Marketed in the 1890s by the Bayer pharmaceutical firm in Germany – Felix Hoffmann, a chemist at the company, was searching for a treatment for his father's arthritis – aspirin was aimed at the control of pain, inflammation and fever. It was certainly not an invented molecule, for it had been known from ancient times that willow bark (from which aspirin was developed) had medicinal properties. In the mid-1700s, a Reverend Edmund Stone had reported to the British Royal Society that because willow bark tasted to him like quinine, he had tried it on fifty patients with painful and debilitating rheumatoid arthritis; all, he claimed, had benefited. It was used increasingly in the nineteenth century until the means were developed to isolate aspirin (salicylic acid), manufacture it in sufficiently large quantities and then market it commercially.

Meanwhile, techniques of drug production were emerging. A way to mass-produce sugar-coated pills was developed in France, and a tablet-compression machine was introduced in England; pharmaceutical companies like Squibb, Eli Lilly and Parke-Davis were founded in the United States and were provided with a sad stimulus to manufacture and market drugs by the American Civil War. Purified forms of ether and chloroform made anaesthesia safer, and plant products were analysed to isolate morphine for systemic pain control and cocaine for local pain. Indeed, one might think of the late nineteenth century as the first phase of modern pharmacology, the phase of pain control.

If so, the first half of the twentieth century would be the phase of infection control. Unlike the agents of pain control, medicines for infectious disease could fairly be seen as allies in a battle; the hordes of microbes assaulting the body seemed a tangible enemy. Ehrlich fired the first shot with his Salvarsan, and quinine derivatives were extensively used in malaria, while arsenic and other toxic elements continued to be used against tropical parasitic diseases. But it was not until the 1930s that Gerhard Domagk, a research director for the Bayer company, discovered that a new fabric dye contained the first true chemotherapy agent – sulfanilamide – a drug that hindered germs while having very few adverse effects on the body. As in Ehrlich's dream, it targeted bacteria and prevented them from multiplying, giving the body a needed chance to mount its own defences. Among the infectious scourges treatable with it and related 'sulfa' drugs were puerperal or childbed fever, meningitis and most pneumonias, all of which had often been deadly since ancient times.

Penicillin was even more powerful. Identified in 1928 by Alexander Fleming and developed in the 1930s by Howard Florey and Ernst Chain, it came into widespread use during the Second World War. It dramatically improved survival from battle wound infections, as well as curing many cases of syphilis among soldiers – a magic bullet apparently as penetrating and accurate as any Paul Ehrlich had dreamed of. In 1944 Selman Waxman, a microbiologist who was an expert on funguses in soil, discovered streptomycin, a component of one such fungus, which appeared to be effective against the tubercle bacillus – the killer of countless TB sufferers for centuries. The British Medical Research Council, after several years of clinical trials, announced in 1948 that they had 'the clearest possible proof' that acute, progressive tuberculosis, the most devastating kind, 'could be halted by streptomycin'.

The rising prestige of medicine throughout the half-century since has been built on this enthusiasm for 'miracle cures'. Not only drug treatment but surgery too received an immense boost from antibiotics, just as it had from ether; all too frequently until then, skilful surgery was doomed by infection. Dramatic books and movies recounted the stories of the 'microbe hunters' – heroes who were almost as luminous as the victorious Allied commanders. Although these were heroes of the laboratory, the white-coated men (there were few women doctors then) in the clinics and hospital wards found that the lustre rubbed off on them. Knowing how and when to fire the magic bullets against bacteria made them into knights in shining armour.

But chinks had already appeared in that armour. The first dose of penicillin injected into a patient had been given in January 1941. Only about a year later, in early 1942, doctors found strains of bacteria that resisted penicillin. It *should* have targeted them. They were staphylococci, the same wound-infecting species that had been dramatically susceptible a year before. Yet not only were they resistant, but they appeared regularly in hospitals by the early 1950s, spreading through patients and hospital staff alike.

By 1946 strains of gonorrhoea resistant to penicillin had emerged and began to spread. By 1960 doctors in Britain had to use doses fifty times the original ones to combat these new microbes, and by 1980 the doses required with some strains were simply intolerable. Syphilis, Paul Ehrlich's old nemesis, also arose in resistant strains. By the 1970s sexually transmitted diseases thought by many to have been conquered rode the wave of sexual permissiveness to new epidemic heights. And in the 1980s minor or even obscure viruses, not susceptible to antibiotics in the first place – hepatitis, herpes and the dreaded AIDS – overtook a chastened and saddened human consciousness.

The 'restless tide' was a phrase used by Doctor Richard Krause – then Director of America's National Institute of Allergy and Infectious Diseases, and since winner of the coveted Koch prize for research on microbes – to describe the way these tiny organisms keep coming back at us. As an ocean shore is continually disturbed by waves, they recede for a while, and may lull the unsuspecting into a secure reverie, but they always return in one form or another to beat against the poorly protected shores of our health and safety. Only a crafty vigilance proves responsive enough to their vagaries, and even such vigilance is often not enough, so that we find ourselves surprised, repairing damage that had not been anticipated.

Consider the change of metaphors for the microbes that cause disease: for Paul Ehrlich, a tangible enemy that could be named and targeted with our hoped-for magic bullets – a war that could eventually be won once and for all; for Richard Krause, a restless, nameless tide surging endlessly at our boundaries, predictable only in its eternal recurrences. If Ehrlich had contemplated his Darwin – *The Origin of Species* had been published when he was a child – he might have guessed what would happen. Microbes, like all forms of life, are constantly evolving, adapting to new conditions that the environment presents to them. Penicillin did not spell doom for the streptococcus and gonococcus; it merely presented them with an unusual evolutionary challenge. In the end the microbes could almost be seen to be thumbing their noses at us; the more pharmacological bullets were fired at them, the more the bacteria adapted – a classic case of an 'evolutionary arms race' between a predator and its prey. As for the virus that causes AIDS, it appears to be an evolutionary novelty – a former monkey virus that evolved the ability to colonize humans – and one that takes full advantage of our many human frailties, not the least of which is the absence of any truly effective anti-viral drug.

Roussel-Uclaf, now part of the international giant Hoechst Roussel, is one of the leading pharmaceutical houses in France, and the one that makes the drug that probably saved James Nelson's life, mifepristone. It was the result of what is known as rational drug development. At its best, this process uses basic chemistry theory about molecular structures to think through to the sort of molecule that is needed for the disease that is being targeted: a molecule that will break through a bacterial wall, say; or in Mr Nelson's case, one that will fit the receptors for cortisol like a hand fitting a glove, but one that will also remain there. Then the tremendous excess of cortisol produced by his tumour would find itself impotent, and the destruction wreaked by it would be repaired. A cure could only be offered by the surgery that ultimately took the tumour away, but in the interim mifepristone worked like a 'designer drug' on the receptors – just as it should, according to the abstract diagrams of chemical theory.

Finding a new and powerful agent against disease was not a new experience for Roussel. In the early decades of the century, and the company's life, it was extensively involved in the production of horse serum, and scores of horses were stabled at the company to be injected with microbes and later bled. This activity was based in part on a scientific concept: horses or other animals would raise their own antibodies to the microbes, and their serum, carrying these antibodies, could help fight off dangerous microbes in the bloodstream of a critically ill person. This system is still in use in one situation today: a bite from a snake that carries venom toxic to nerves can kill a person quickly, but injection with anti-venom – serum from horses exposed to the venom – is often life-saving.

However, horse serum, including the relatively pure form used against snake-bites today, occasionally causes an overwhelming systemic collapse called anaphylactic shock – total body reaction as deadly as any microbe or venom. Roussel also marketed a non-specific form of horse serum as a tonic – an example of over-marketing of a type that has unfortunately been repeated in various ways by many drug companies since – but even in the specific case of microbes, the early twentieth-century serum produced by Roussel and others simply did not work well enough even when shock was avoided.

The advent of antibiotics changed all that. According to Edouard Sakiz, a chemist who heads the company, the modern era at Roussel-Uclaf began when it purchased a company called Sofrapen (Société Française de Pénicilline). Demand for its product grew rapidly during the Second World War and thereafter, establishing the company as a major presence in the pharmaceutical industry's increasingly international market.

But this energetic production and distribution of penicillin, which was engaged in by a number of firms and a great many doctors, almost immediately began to generate resistant strains of microbes – the adaptive rising again of the 'restless tide'. Patients were being hospitalized and were dying once more of pneumonias and other infections that had seemed completely curable a few years earlier. Understanding of the evolutionary realities of bacterial growth dawned on doctors and scientists, and the search for new and different antibiotics intensified. Bacteria were adapting to penicillin's action; this made it essential to understand what that action was, and to develop new kinds of antibiotics that did not just mimic penicillin's mode of attack, but rather used a different chemical tactic or strategy.

In retrospect, it seemed to Sakiz as if he and his colleagues at Roussel were engaged in an endless war. It turned out that the way penicillin fought bacteria was to throw a chemical spanner into their machinery for building protective walls around themselves. Resistance to penicillin was eventually understood to come from bacteria that could manufacture their own retaliatory weapon, an enzyme that was called penicillinase because it broke down and destroyed penicillin. Streptomycin, the next antibiotic to be developed after penicillin, used a new strategy: it interfered with the bacteria's protein-making machinery. But this action made it dangerously toxic to patients in the long run.

Eventually, in 1980/81, a new weapon was produced: cefotaxime, a molecule that the company marketed under the name Claforan. This was one of a general category of new drugs that used the same strategy as penicillin – preventing bacteria from making their own protective walls – but added a new tactic: a molecular shield against penicillinase. Thus many bacteria that could destroy penicillin were helpless against Claforan. Roussel had invented a decisive new weapon, one still in use today, and there have been many other new agents developed in response to the adaptive challenges constantly offered by microbes; Roussel itself is presently working on a new antibiotic more powerful than Claforan. In the best medical centres, these newer, more potent agents are guarded closely and kept for situations where all else has been tried and has failed. Such restricted use can greatly lengthen the time it takes for bacteria to evolve, adapt and resist a new agent.

But resistance will still develop eventually. Ironically, the most intractable infections are acquired by patients in hospitals. These 'noso-comial' diseases – *nosocomium* is a Greek word for hospital – develop most readily where antibiotics are extensively used. In effect the modern hospital is a focal point of bacterial evolution. Here, the microbes face the most secret weapons of the medical care army, the newest, most penetrating 'magic bullets', and in time they 'learn' to deal with them.

But ordinary people – you and I – walking into the doctor's surgery are as much to blame as anyone for the rise of resistant microbes. It is we who, throughout the 1950s and 1960s, and to a lesser extent thereafter, have pressured doctors to give us antibiotics for ordinary colds, stomach viruses and 'flu' – viral conditions for which antibiotics are useless. Since all of us are constantly colonized by bacteria, includ-ing some that in larger numbers cause illness, every time we take a course of penicillin or erythromycin we don't need, we turn our own bodies into little laboratories for the breeding of resistant germs. And widespread use of antibiotics in livestock exacerbates the problem.

Because restrictions on the sale of antibiotics are much looser in the developing world, where the drugs are often sold over the counter, the development of resistance has been a greater problem there. Amer-ican men and women serving in the Gulf War, for example, contracted bacterial forms of diarrhoea that proved resistant to a distressingly wide range of antibiotics. And the more resistance there is, the more money pharmaceutical companies invest in new antibiotic research – money that they then recoup, as well as gleaning hefty profits from, by charging very high prices for the very newest drugs. Centoxin, a new agent for resistant septic shock – a life-threatening cardiovascular collapse caused by bacteria spread in hospitals – is made through the latest techniques of biotechnology. It works very well, and it clearly saves lives. But it costs some £2000 a dose.

Jarrow, across the river from Newcastle in the north-east of England, is an industrial community that has experienced in microcosm the cycle of success and failure of antibiotics throughout the developed world. Doctors George Grant and David Gregory have been in general practice there for more than four decades, and Grant can also draw on his physician-father's experience before him. During the 1930s severe unemployment produced poverty on a scale that invited infectious disease, with inadequate medical care that few of the poor could anyway afford. Grant recalls that in the immediate post-war period, when the National Health Service was introduced, Jarrow had the highest rate of tuberculosis in Britain, and he vividly remembers the impact of the first use of streptomycin.

One of his patients, Mary Harding, was a young married woman with a new baby when she was hospitalized with 'a particularly virulent, bad form of tuberculosis'. As Grant reminded her forty years later, 'You were very ill, and practically everybody who had that condition died – until 1950, when this wonder drug, streptomycin, was invented.' Mary Harding had an injection of streptomycin every day for 150 days. 'After four injections, I felt really ... well, alive. Once I started on that streptomycin, I could've come home if they would've let me.' Doctor Grant had been taught as a medical student that nobody recovered from such a virulent case of tuberculosis. But he and her other physicians had been alert enough to give her this brand-new agent, streptomycin, and four decades later he was chatting with her about her grandchildren.

To Grant, streptomycin was 'even more dramatic than the invention of penicillin, which had preceded it, because this was a chronic condition ... and it was marvellous.' But by 1955 tuberculosis had become resistant to streptomycin, so that doses had to be increased to levels that could cause deafness. Combination drug regimens began to be used, and soon streptomycin was replaced by a new two-drug treatment programme. Drug company scientists were already caught up in their race against bacterial evolution, and by the 1960s antibiotics had created a multibillion-pound market worldwide.

In 1989 Marjorie Jobling, a patient of Doctor Gregory's in her forties, faced a situation not very different from that of Mary Harding forty years earlier. A sufferer from asthma for many years, she developed a severe chest ailment – not in itself life-threatening. 'Asthmatics do tend to develop chest infections. We went to see her on a call, and she was pretty ill, but she clearly had an infection. So I put her on amoxycillin, which is a standard broad-spectrum penicillin, and that didn't seem to work. So I changed it to erythromycin, which is the usual treatment for less typical infections causing pneumonia, and it's almost guaranteed to clear them up. But in fact that didn't work either.'

Marjorie continued to decline for three weeks, and eventually, after she had been sleepless and hallucinating for eight days, she was hospitalized, where the same two drugs were tried again, without success. 'They put her on a very old antibiotic that's been around a long time – chloramphenicol – which is considered rather dangerous. It can produce some blood side-effects.' These can be devastating, but fortunately they did not occur in this case and the drug cured Marjorie Jobling's pneumonia.

Doctor Grant and Doctor Gregory struggle constantly, in general practice, to keep abreast of the restless bacterial tide. At the same time they must negotiate the shoals of drug-company marketing, with its confusing array of 'me-too' drugs – drugs that are virtually the same but all marketed under different names – and with high-pressure sales techniques that sometimes verge on bribery. Drug companies in the United States, for example, spend thousands of dollars per doctor per year to bring their message to practitioners. Yet Spanish physicians prescribe twice as many antibiotics as Americans, and Germany has been called 'the last Garden of Eden' for the drug companies. Concern about this illogical variation has led Doctors Grant and Gregory to serve on an international panel trying to rationalize prescribing. Given the many pressures from patients, drug company representatives and even scientists enthusiastic about their latest discoveries, a doctor in practice must have not only good judgement but great strength of character, as well as energy to wade through the literature, to adjust the prescribing regimen in a way that is best for the patient, especially in the many cases where no one is really sure what the best regimen is.

Antibiotics, important as they have been, are only one category of drugs. Others are pain-killers, anti-cancer drugs, heart drugs and blood pressure drugs, to name just a few. Each without exception raises the red flag of risk to one degree or another, because none has a perfectly focused range of effects. Every prescription is in fact a balancing of risks. In the case of cancer drugs a process almost analogous to bacterial evolution goes on inside the body as susceptible tumour cells fall by the wayside and resistant ones come to the fore. Even when the drugs are successful they have a wide range of unwanted effects. Cancer is essentially runaway cell growth. Drugs that work interfere with the production of new cells, which means they prevent not only new cancer cells from forming but also new cells in normal organs. Thus the devastating effects they can have on blood cells, on hair growth and on the lining of the gut. In a sad irony, some of them are also to some degree cancer-causing agents themselves.

But this classification-by-purpose – heart drugs, tumour drugs, etc. – is too crude for physicians and scientists, who must also know the kind of chemical structure a drug has. Analysis of this structure will eventually lead to an understanding of how it works, and then to the rational crafting of new and even more useful molecules. One such category is the steroids, a group of molecules with great biological importance.

Among the naturally occurring ones are the main sex hormones of women and men, oestrogen and testosterone; the pregnancy hormone, progesterone; and the 'fight or flight' stress hormone, cortisol. All are more or less flat molecules made up of four rings and consisting mostly of carbon. They vary in function as atoms of carbon, oxygen and hydrogen are added to or removed from the four-ring lattice. In size, these molecules are middling – far larger than a molecule of table salt, but tiny compared to proteins like insulin. The body's own steroids are all made from cholesterol, a dangerous substance in excess, but at lower levels essential for body functioning.

Artificial steroids now number in the thousands, but in the late 1940s techniques of making them were just being worked out. Understanding of their structure came mainly from study of the adrenal gland. Physicians and scientists at the Mayo Clinic in Rochester, Minnesota, managed to synthesize cortisone, a modified form of the adrenal gland's own cortisol hormone. This manufactured agent proved to combat inflammation, just as the natural hormone does. When they gave it to patients with rheumatoid arthritis – a crippling, excruciatingly painful condition – some who had been confined to their beds in contorted positions for years were able to flex their limbs again. A Nobel Prize for some of the scientists in 1950 recognized this series of accomplishments.

Here, apparently, was a miracle drug that worked not against an infectious microbe but against a derangement of the body's own processes. Unfortunately the effects of cortisone on arthritis were not permanent, but a bridge had been crossed into a scientific region full of new possibilities. The lesson was not lost on the pharmaceutical industry, where many companies geared up for turning out new steroid molecules. Powerful new ones were effective for inflammation, head injury and disorders of the adrenal gland, such as that of James Nelson.

Chemical mastery of this family of molecules had enormous implications for other body systems, in particular the ones in each sex that control reproduction. Drugs with potential for the treatment of infertility, lack of sexual desire, menstrual disorders and problems of pregnancy were being developed. One of the earliest of these was synthesized in Britain in 1938 by Charles Dodds, and slowly gained currency as a treatment for women who had trouble maintaining a pregnancy. There was a plausible theory behind it: the drug, diethylstilbestrol, or DES, was a synthetic oestrogen, and oestrogen was one of the main hormones of pregnancy. Some poor, uncontrolled studies at the time seemed to show that it worked.

Later controlled studies showed that it did not work, but by then millions of normal women had been given the drug during pregnancy in the belief that it might be helpful. Tragically, a small proportion of the girls to whom those women gave birth – somewhere between one in ten thousand and one in a thousand of all women exposed to the drug – grew up to develop a previously rare and often deadly cancer of the vagina. At best, these women were forced in their teens or twenties to chose between their reproductive organs and their lives, since only radical surgery had a chance of saving them. Fortunately they have so far only numbered in the hundreds, and the drug is no longer in use. Candice Tedeschi, a nurse at the Long Island Jewish Hospital in New York, runs a clinic devoted to DES victims. She knows the drug's dangers as well as anyone, but can speak in a surprisingly balanced way about them:

> We don't call it the practice of medicine for nothing. It *is* practice. We are human, we are not perfect, we make mistakes. And this mistake of DES was a combination mistake, between the drug companies and the medical profession, so blindly accepting this drug and giving it so widely. Here on the East Coast they gave this drug to almost everybody. I have doctors here who gave it to almost every single pregnant woman who walked in – not because they had any particular problem, but to make normal pregnancies more normal.

Few people would suggest that we wait twenty or more years to see the ultimate results of a new drug before using it. But this drug was a needless one, not unlike thalidomide, a non-steroid tranquillizer that in the 1960s caused severe birth defects when given to pregnant women to help with distressing but not life-threatening morning sickness. Thalidomide together with the artificial oestrogen DES had the effect of changing drastically the way doctors and scientists prescribe drugs for pregnant women.

By far the most important steroids connected with the reproductive system – indeed, the most momentous pharmacological discoveries of the 1950s – were, however, the agents that had the power to prevent unwanted births. These oral contraceptives, mostly steroids or molecules resembling steroids, began to provide women and their partners with decisive choice about when to conceive. Although like all drugs they had a 'down side' – increasing the risk of stroke, for example – there is no doubt that the formulations used today are remarkably safe and effective when properly prescribed and used.

However, these drugs had another, much broader religious and social dimension. Vigorous opposition from the Catholic Church and some other religious groups threatened the whole concept of artificial birth control. As Edouard Sakiz recalls it, Roussel-Uclaf had been well positioned scientifically and organizationally to make a major contribution to this 'classical' period of birth control drugs, partly because of its experience with steroids. But Sakiz's boss at the time frustrated his efforts completely because of religious opposition to birth control. For perhaps the first time new drug development was being influenced not just by medical and scientific considerations but by powerful cultural factors (although even Salvarsan had had its opponents, who thought treating syphilis would encourage sexual licence). Sakiz always regretted this lost opportunity, and when he took over as head of the company he promised himself that future chances like it would not be passed up.

By this time a highly creative physician-scientist, Etienne-Emile Baulieu, was involved in steroid hormone studies at the French national medical research institute, and had worked out some very fundamental facts about how these molecules affect cells. Georges Teutsch and other scientists at Roussel, like Ehrlich in an earlier era, were generating thousands upon thousands of compounds in the hope of finding active and safe new agents. Baulieu collaborated with them in an attempt to make a safe and effective analogue of progesterone, the hormone that promotes fertility and helps maintain pregnancy. The result was a new molecule that blocked progesterone powerfully. Compounds at the company labs were given the RU tag, for Roussel-Uclaf, and a number; this one was designated RU 38 486 – or for short, RU 486.

RU 486 was soon shown to be safe in monkey studies, and then was shown to be effective in bringing an early end to pregnancy in nine out of eleven women who requested an abortion early in pregnancy. By 1992, a little over a decade after research had created the new molecule, around a hundred thousand women in France alone had received the drug, in combination with a well-known agent called a prostaglandin, given two days later. This treatment had proved very safe, with only three women per hundred experiencing unsuccessful or incomplete abortion (easily completed with surgery) and less than one per cent excessive bleeding. This rate of success compares very favourably with that of the far more onerous procedure of surgical abortion.

By 1988 gynaecologists, family planners and women generally were hailing RU 486 as an enormous medical advance, in effect a magic bullet for unwanted early pregnancy. But the company received hundreds of letters from anti-abortion groups and individuals who considered the drug a 'death pill'. Some would later compare Etienne-Emile Baulieu – by then a member of the extremely prestigious National Academy of Sciences of the United States and an obvious candidate for a Nobel Prize – to Adolf Hitler. Threats of boycott of all the company's drugs, some vastly more important commercially than RU 486, led Roussel to withdraw the drug from the French market in late 1988.

But as luck would have it, the World Congress of Obstetrics and Gynaecology was meeting in Rio de Janiero at the time, and Baulieu was speaking there. The company soon received a petition bearing the signatures of hundreds of experts and practitioners in reproductive medicine threatening a boycott of their own, and demanding that the drug be released again. Those who signed included many who stood to lose income if surgical abortion were to be replaced by a drug; clearly their protest was not selfishly motivated. On account of the French government's financial interest in the company, Claude Evin, the health minister of France, became involved. He soon put an end to Roussel's indecision and ordered the drug back on the market, threatening among other things to give the patent away. He justified his decision by saying he 'could not permit the abortion debate to deprive women of a product that represents medical progress'. RU 486 was 'la propriété morale des femmes françaises' – the moral property of women, not just the property of the drug company.

Baulieu, who often says 'I am a medical doctor who does science', fully agreed, and he has interrupted much of his science to be an advocate for the drug. He recalls his early, impressionable days in medicine when – at the age of eighteen or nineteen – the suffering of patients affected him permanently. He describes the desperate situation he saw in India, where population explosion produced widespread disease and death in childhood. And he rarely fails to mention the two hundred thousand deaths a year worldwide – 'one every three minutes' – of women who have suffered botched abortions. The father of three and grandfather of seven, he would like to see unwanted birth stopped, not in spite of his love for children but in part because of it. Largely due to his leadership, France, a Catholic country with a potentially vigorous opposition and a long medical tradition strongly favouring motherhood, has become the undisputed world leader in the pharmaceutical termination of unwanted pregnancy. Britain lags behind, but is moving, while the United States has not yet awakened from its slumber.

Like pro-choice people throughout the world, the French consider legal abortion the lesser of two evils. Mme Aubény, an experienced nurse who directs a clinic in Paris, has given RU 486 to hundreds of women. She too has her early impressions. 'I remember one of the first times I ever came in the hospital, I saw a twenty-year-old woman die from a failed abortion. And a little later there was a thirty-five-year-old who also died, very painfully, from septicaemia, leaving five children. These are things you never forget, and never want to see again.'

She reflects too on a harsh and inescapable historical reality:

Women have always wanted, since earliest times, to use medicine to produce an abortion. What pills and potions they've taken in this hope! And now at last their wish has come true. We have a drug that can trigger an abortion. But there is another aspect to it that I believe is moral. It's giving back to women some control over their own bodies. In effect, they decide to have an abortion, and *they* supervise it. It's no longer the doctor, the technician, or the surgeon who takes this step. Morally, that's important. It's not a miracle pill; on the contrary, it's a pill that gives great responsibility.

We could scarcely have a better demonstration of the fact that medical science does not exist in a social vacuum, but on the contrary is stimulated, buffeted and sometimes blocked by what anthropologists call the 'social construction' of scientific advances – a fancy way of referring to what people in a culture collectively think the advance means. RU 486 is now licensed for use in Britain, Scandinavia, China, and elsewhere, but it is not even permitted to be *tested* for pregnancy termination in the United States, because of the well-organized and vocal anti-abortion minority in that country. This minority could damage the market of any pharmaceutical firm in America that even begins to test it. Although states such as New York and California have been trying to circumvent these obstacles, the present government in Washington is highly unlikely to be of any help.

Sadly, this has implications far beyond the abortion issue. As Baulieu points out, the ideal fate of a new drug is to take advantage of multiple targets and uses of the same molecule. The very problem of unwanted effects of a powerful agent – the fact that it goes to various cells and combines with different receptors – also provides an enormous opportunity. The steroid hormone system that Baulieu has spent his life studying makes it possible for RU 486 to be used in a number of different medical settings. Not only does it have other obstetric uses – promoting expulsion of an already dead foetus that is endangering the mother, for example, and stimulating labour so that a woman who is past term can give birth to a normal baby – it is also being tested in Montpellier, in the south of France, as a treatment for breast cancer, and it shows great promise. Physicians in Holland and elsewhere are testing it against certain brain tumours that are promoted by progesterone. And in Finland researchers are experimenting with it as a conventional contraceptive.

Even in the United States some research teams are testing the drug in cases of glaucoma and advanced breast cancer. But the most successful American test so far has been for the illness that James Nelson had, Cushing's Syndrome. That is because RU 486 blocks not only progesterone receptors but also, in higher doses, receptors for cortisol, the body hormone that Mr Nelson had in devastating excess. RU 486 is, by another name, mifepristone, the drug that Mr Nelson got from Doctor Nieman in an experimental programme at the National Institutes of Health in Washington, and the drug that in all likelihood saved his life.

Although the 'magic bullet' notion originated with Ehrlich, the focus on microbes as a singular cause of infectious disease preceded him by several decades. One of the most dominant ideas in nineteenth-century medicine had been that *social* conditions foster disease. Hygienists – today we would call them public health workers – repeatedly showed that people living in bad social and economic conditions were much more vulnerable to the great infectious scourges that still assaulted the world. Millions in Europe and the United States lived in overcrowded conditions without effective toilets, running water or fresh air, and ate food from unsupervised markets that were frequently contaminated. Although the notion of microscopic creatures causing disease had been discussed for a long time, it was still considered fanciful, and many thoughtful people who looked at the statistics saw strong evidence that most disease was caused by poverty and the social life that was tied to it.

Their work was known as the sanitary movement, or the social hygiene movement, and they believed that disease would never be effectively combated without great changes in society. Rudolph Virchow of Germany is known to physicians as the 'father of pathology' and one of the greatest of all medical scientists. But he was also an extremely active social hygienist throughout his life, and even supported the revolutions of 1848 because he believed it his duty as a doctor to change the social conditions that cause disease. 'Don't we see,' he wrote, 'that epidemics everywhere point to deficiencies of society?'

Half a century later, even after the dawn of modern drug research, the great Russian playwright Anton Chekhov – who was also a physician, calling medicine his wife and literature his mistress – did a health survey of the island of Sakhalin off Siberia, where convicts and their families lived under dismal conditions. By this time such surveys were fairly common, although usually closer to home. Chekhov saw the Sakhalin survey as discharging his 'debt to medicine' – in other words, as part of the responsibility of a doctor. In three months he interviewed almost everyone on the island, and drew a conclusion: servitude, whippings, alcohol abuse, prostitution and poverty combined to produce inevitable disease. The social hygiene viewpoint of Virchow still seemed valid to Chekhov at the dawn of the twentieth century.

But between Virchow's youthful activism and Chekhov's principled voyage, there was half a century of changing medical thought. Pasteur had established the germ theory – ancient but not accepted – on a firm scientific foundation. Claude Bernard, also in France, had founded the field of experimental physiology as a testing ground for medical theory. And Virchow himself, in his role as a clinical and postmortem pathologist, had promoted the concept of disease entities – systematically known processes that could be clearly identified from their paths of destruction in the body. These three currents of thought came together in the ideas of Robert Koch, who devised a paradigm for the interpretation of disease. In this method, a microscopic organism had to be identified, then located in the diseased organs and finally shown to be capable of causing the disease in an experimental animal. What, a few decades earlier, had been a complex result of social, economic and cultural conditions was now seen as an attack by a singular microbe – one type for each disease, strong but not invincible.

The stage was set for Paul Ehrlich, working on syphilis, to imagine his 'silver bullet'. No longer was it necessary to moralize about prostitution and promiscuity, as the religious branch of the sanitary movement eagerly did, or to point out how poverty and middle-class marital customs – husbands frequenting prostitutes while wives looked the other way – contributed to the disease's spread. Now there was a new approach: magic bullet against nefarious microbe. This was fine as far as it went – and something of both its success and its limitations has already been mentioned in terms of side-effects and the evolution of resistance. But even more important than these is an indirect result of the magic-bullet viewpoint: the neglect of all the conditions that make life easy for the microbe and also weaken the body's stance against invasion.

These are the same social and economic conditions Virchow had understood during the revolutions of 1848. While Ehrlich was inching his way towards Salvarsan at the turn of the century, Chekhov was dying of tuberculosis. He knew quite well that among his fellow sufferers were a disproportionate number of the poor, and he established a sanitarium for their care before he died. But what he could not have forseen was that effective treatment would elude physicians for another half century and that during that time – between 1900 and 1950 – tuberculosis would decline enormously because of improving social conditions. When George Grant talks about his physician-father in Jarrow battling this same disease in the depths of the 1930s Depression, he does not mention that social conditions had been much worse in earlier decades, that TB had already been enormously reduced and that vast numbers of lives had been saved, and would continue to be saved, by social, not medical, intervention. Today TB is rising again fast, for many of the same reasons, especially among the poorest communities in the United States.

What had always been true of infectious disease was also increasingly true of other, newer diseases, like the ones the young doctors at Johns Hopkins were struggling against. Heart attack, stroke, chronic lung disease and several major cancers rose dramatically in our century, and they have proved to be more common in the poor. Poverty today brings with it lack of access to timely medical care, as well as abuse of cigarettes, alcohol, street drugs and food, not to mention prostitution and violence – all major routes to current deaths among the poor. Yet ironically the Hopkins doctors, and their patients as well, are still burdened by the 'one disease, one microbe' magic bullet approach to treatment. The quick fix that was insufficient for infectious disease does not even begin to be appropriate for chronic disease of the sort we have today. The social conditions that helped cause the nineteenth-century scourges are at least equally implicated in our own twentieth-century ones. And that is why Reverend Tuggle may be making more headway against them from his pulpit or in the basement of his church than the Hopkins doctors do in their high-tech hospital.

Baulieu himself, for whom Ehrlich is a hero, says 'I don't like very much the word magic bullet. Number one, I don't like bullet, because I'm rather pacifist. And number two, magic – I don't like magic. Because what we are doing in fact is, in humanistic terms, a rational approach of nature. And there is no space for magic.' When he thinks about RU 486, he does not imagine a quick fix, not least because pregnancy is not a disease. He knows that the culture of poverty is partly responsible for deaths from abortions and for unwanted, starving children, but he sees no point in sermonizing to women about sex, especially to those who are already pregnant. So he invented a tool for women to use right now, a stopgap measure in the war against botched abortions, until that imagined future day when all people are prudent, until the world becomes a substantially better place.

Few people anywhere in the world today doubt the power of the profit motive in unleashing human energies, and that applies to drug development as much as to anything else. It is very unlikely that a government-sponsored steroid hormone research programme could produce and screen 38 486 molecules – the number screened by Roussel – in search of a few effective ones. The billions of pounds that drug companies make from the world market buy some expensive lunches, to be sure, but they also pay the salaries of thousands of scientists and the upkeep of their laboratories. Many of these scientists have discovered extremely valuable drugs and some, like Gertrude Elion, have won the Nobel Prize for truly exceptional contributions – in her case for work on anti-cancer drugs. Government cannot support all the needed research on drugs and the annual budget of the private sector is several times that of the entire National Institutes of Health in the United States, the Medical Research Council in Britain and other public research-funding agencies. We cannot move forward in this kind of research without the profit motive – the greed, if you like – of investors in pharmaceutical firms around the world.

But in accepting this necessity, we must also realize that it carries risks. Candice Tedeschi, who has spent many years identifying and caring for the victims of DES, says, 'I don't want to come across negative against drugs ... Drugs are wonderful things that we need desperately in our world, to help us have long, healthy, productive lives. But we have to have some sort of control over [them]. *Is the drug doing more good than it's doing harm?*'

A large proportion of the most frequently prescribed drugs for the elderly, major consumers of drugs, are misprescribed; they either should not be given for the condition in question, or there are better drugs or other treatments for the same problem. According to Doctor Sidney Wolfe, who represents a Washington public interest group that evaluates drugs for consumers, a large proportion are dangerous; 104 of the 287 most frequently prescribed drugs, for example, are deemed by his assessment to be too dangerous for people over sixty-five to use. Many more are of questionable value, or duplicate at greater expense the effects of older drugs.

The avidity of drug company salespeople, the aggression of their advertising and the financially competitive rather than public-spirited nature of their activities exacerbate misprescribing, and in some countries with over-the-counter sales they bypass physicians altogether. The thousands of pounds, dollars, francs or yen spent by the firms every year to bring their at best biased message to each physician make objective medical decision-making difficult.

In a fascinating study published in the *Annals of Internal Medicine* in June 1992, Doctor Michael Wilkes and his colleagues at UCLA examined 109 full-page pharmaceutical advertisements in ten leading US medical journals. The ads were sent to more than a hundred medical scientists and more than fifty pharmacists, all highly experienced in evaluating research in the areas relevant to the ad. Although pharmaceutical advertising is in general far more accurate than non-medical advertising, more than half the ads were judged by at least two out of three reviewers to be misleading enough to have been rejected outright by the journal or accepted only after major revision. And more than ninety per cent of the ads were judged by reviewers to violate the advertising standards laid down by the FDA in at least one minor or major way.

Misprescribing, including unnecessary prescribing and the failure to use generic substitutes, is a major factor in the widely recognized waste of health care funds. In Britain the government is now attempting to reduce such costs by asking GPs to prescribe only the cheaper substitutes and introducing financial incentives for GP practices to keep within recommended budgets by limiting the prescription of costly rare drugs. In the United States a network of illegal pharmacies has grown up around AIDS victims, creating a black market in useless and dangerous illegal drugs. And in Spain – as in countries all over the world – some pharmacists, dismayed by bloated drug-company claims, have turned in frustration to untested herbal remedies. While some of these ancient nostrums may prove useful, others will no doubt turn out to be useless or quite harmful; just as with commercial drugs, only scientific research can determine which is which. Any plan for health care at the national level has to include attempts to reduce all this uncertainty and waste, and rationalize the bewildering alternatives.

Some of our expectations as consumers are exaggerated and irrational as well. People demand more stringent controls on manu-factured drugs, yet they also go to herbalists seeking substances subject to no standards of purity and never properly tested at all. (One such seemingly harmless 'natural' substance, tryptophan, which was sold over-the-counter in health food stores, caused a small epidemic of serious muscle disease because of impurities in the preparation. People demand that no new drugs be marketed unless proved conclusively to be both useful and safe; yet the AIDS patients' movement in the US – where new drug evaluation has long been more stringent than in Europe – requested and then essentially forced the FDA to release several major new drugs without leaving time for legally mandated testing. Ironically, the search for an AIDS vaccine is being held back by drug manufacturers' fears of lawsuits that may follow testing – a situation that puts the AIDS vaccine in a growing category of new or proposed drugs that are 'orphaned' because public demands for drug safety have reached such an exaggerated and threatening pitch. Medi-cine cannot be all things to all people; we must decide for ourselves what risks we are willing to take in order to reap the potential benefits of drug development.

Yet more important, perhaps, is the lulling effect of dream drugs. In the minds of many people there are, or soon will be, magic bullets for every disease or complaint. In this tragically mistaken belief we cease to think about our own responsibility and blithely go on with the behaviours and habits that bring on disease or make it worse. In East Africa there is a myth that AIDS can now be cured, a myth apparently centred on an experimental and untested drug called Kemron, developed in Kenya; millions of people may contract the virus and die because they are soothed by this belief. But such an attitude is not restricted to places like Africa; we go through an almost identical process in the West.

In the last few years we have heard that new drugs can reverse the atherosclerosis – fatty thickening – that clogs the arteries and leads to heart attack or stroke. So we reach for the extra cream puff or the 'juicy' steak with subconscious confidence that whatever harm it may do to us can be fixed later on. We have heard too that the new gene technology methods will revolutionize cancer treatment, so millions of us go on smoking with the tacit assumption that lung cancer will be curable by the time we get it. These mental processes are as primitive as any in Africa, and far less excusable, since we have access to information that most Africans do not.

We may need to reverse in part the process we went through in the second half of the nineteenth century, when the hygiene movement was replaced by the aggressive modern focus on microbes. This was before the rise of heart disease, stroke and cancer as the greatest killers. Back then, it seemed simple: each major deadly disease had its very own microbe-cause; identify it, find its weak point, destroy it – end of disease. But of the most dangerous ailments in the Western world today, only AIDS has a good chance of one day (and not soon) being preventable by vaccine; none of these illnesses has a good chance of a pharmacological cure. The drugs that work are messy, dangerous and only partly effective.

Yet we can do things now that would reduce mortality from these major killers by millions of deaths a year – or at a minimum postpone those deaths until very old age. And most of our options have to do with social conditions and cultural habits. In the previous chapter it was shown how the social conditions of East Baltimore, including lack of access to timely medical care, foster advanced and incurable chronic illnesses. But is this really like nineteenth-century poverty fostering infectious scourges through malnutrition and lack of sanitation?

In a word, yes. Self-abusive habits target human vulnerability just as surely as microbes do. The vulnerability of the poor has three separate components. The first is lack of information. Everyone knows, for example, that cigarettes are coffin nails, but as advertisers are well aware, information must sink in – it must be repeated again and again in different contexts, and be supported by expert advice and colloquial word of mouth. That is why more highly educated people are less likely to be smokers and why doctors and nurses have very low rates of the habit. Poor people are exposed to far more disinformation about cigarettes, through advertising and word of mouth, than to information. And the truth is not reinforced by the milieu. Similar arguments can be made about alcohol, cocaine, heroin, dangerous foods with high levels of saturated fat, even high-risk sex.

The second component of vulnerability is the tremendous incentive that draws people towards these habits and addictions. Consider how well-meaning advice must strike impoverished people: *You mean, in the midst of all this misery, you want me to give up the one thing I really enjoy? You must be kidding.* A pleasurable healthy lifestyle with a comfortable home in a safe neighbourhood, good-quality food and leisure activities like sports and gym workouts costs money that these people do not have. So they turn to the pleasures that *are* available to them, and for a time at least they really do enjoy them.

Finally, all this is compounded by the lack of disincentives. The concept that you may be sick ten or twenty years from now if you don't stop your X-Y-Z is relevant for those who can envisage a decent future. But for people who can see no future other than one filled with the same misery as the present, there is no good reason to make a serious effort to reach it. It is this lack of hope that may be the most damaging social condition of all. Add to this the exuberant heedlessness of youth, and the damage is clearly going to be greatest for the young.

So the solutions of the social hygienists of the mid-1800s are still valid today. As Leon Eisenberg, head of the Department of Social Medicine and Health Policy at the Harvard Medical School, has asked, 'Rudolph Virchow, where are you now that we really need you?' And although dangerous habits are more common among the poor, the rich too indulge in them, and our culture as a whole encourages many of them. As was true in the nineteenth century, and as Virchow said then, disease points to 'deficiencies of society'. Behavioural scientists, epidemiologists, teachers and a few enlightened politicians, journalists and clergy are likely to be the social hygienists of the future. And as we attack the diseases of the present and future, our watchword could well be 'No magic bullet'.

CHAPTER 4

CONCEIVING
the FUTURE

I n Aldous Huxley's novel *Brave New World*, readers of the 1930s were treated to an unsettling vision of the future. The story opens with a tour of the Central London Hatchery and Conditioning Centre, its entrance graced with the motto of the World State: 'Community, Identity, Stability.' We visit the Fertilizing Room, the Bottling Room, the Social Predestination Room. We hear the Director of the Centre discourse on the difficulty of making a large enough number of genetically identical human beings. This difficulty stands in the way of adequate production of lower orders of individuals – Gammas, Deltas and Epsilons – destined for various kinds of menial labour. Only Alphas are permitted to remain unique. In the Hatchery the entire nine months of human gestation take place in test-tubes, and along the way the foetuses are treated with chemicals that will help match them to their destiny in society. After birth, Pavlovian methods of conditioning will continue the shaping process. The human products that emerge at the end will not only be suited to their fated roles in life; they will be positively terrified of departing from those roles. Most amazing of all, they will be happy. Scientific control of human destiny will be total.

It is a chilling vision of a grotesquely over-organized future, yet if Huxley were alive today he might feel we are well on our way to it. At the time of writing this book the first 'test-tube babies' are thirteen years old. Although so far only the very first steps of development can take place outside the womb, and although no one has yet tampered with destiny by altering those steps, thousands of human beings have already begun life 'in glass'. Some eggs, whether in test-tubes or in wombs, have been fertilized by sperm taken from Nobel laureates and other genetic fathers picked with meticulous care. Wombs can be rented, for a price, by those with cash in hand; and frequently their genes travel down the social scale to a womb whose much poorer owner needs the same cash. In addition, at least the last third of gestation can now take place outside the womb, in incubators brimming with up-to-the-moment life-support technology.

We do surgery on other foetuses to correct some of their defects, leaving them to finish gestation inside the womb. Still others we deem unsuitable for survival, and these we remove and dispose of. If a woman is carrying too many foetuses – quintuplets, say – we selectively kill some of them to save the others. We are still far from developing an egg until it becomes a baby, injecting it with this or that to shape it to our visions, but the idea no longer seems like mere science fiction. Later in the growth process, years after birth, we use amphetamines to try to correct hyperactive behaviour, in an effort to create a child who will do better in school. And sometimes growth hormone, now manufactured in DNA factories with unprecedented ease, is used to stimulate growth in shorter than average children who are not at all deficient in the hormone. The idea is simply to make them become taller.

But of all our budding accomplishments, the most remarkable is gene control. We are already deeply engaged in a technological revolution that matches the industrial revolution in importance. The roughly one hundred thousand genes every human being has – each one a string of thousands of life-determining molecules – are being systematically mapped. Some of them have already been manufactured and stored in test-tubes. Others have been experimentally altered in blood cells that have been withdrawn, transformed and returned to their owners – children as well as adults. Still others, at least in animals, have been transformed within fertilized eggs, to be passed on from generation to generation, creating a permanent change in the biological heritage of the organism.

Medically, these methods will be far more important than the magic bullets used by past generations against microbes. Gene control will be our superweapon in the war against cancers, the most feared diseases of our time. Genetic disorders like sickle cell anaemia and cystic fibrosis – biochemical derangements that start at the outset of life with defective genes and proceed to destroy children and young adults slowly and painfully – will become truly manageable for the first time in history. Even diseases caused by microbes may be solved by gene control. The AIDS virus, to take an example, works its effects by invading the genetic machinery of human cells, so an important part of research on AIDS is attempting to understand and control that process. Even some drugs that have nothing directly to do with genes – the insulin needed by some diabetics, for instance – are already being manufactured in a purer form through the same technology of gene control. Those who would stand in the way of this technology are asking us to pay an enormous price in human suffering.

Yet the arguments of such opponents have some ethical and political legitimacy. Today a number of genetic errors can be identified in a man and a woman proposing to marry, and they can be advised of their chances of having a child with the same or a worse defect. Tomorrow perhaps we will forbid them to marry, or even sterilize them. Today it is possible to detect certain abnormalities in the foetus part-way through gestation, and parents can be offered the option of an abortion. Could it be that tomorrow we will require one?

Such scenarios may sound implausible, but as will be seen later in the chapter they already exist in China. Early fears about genetic mutants escaping from gene control laboratories and wreaking havoc in the biological balance of the world – soberly debated in the 1970s and 1980s – have receded in the 1990s and become the stuff of science fiction. But that is far from saying that serious abuses are unlikely to happen. When we are able to peer into and tinker with the basic machinery that makes us what we are, such fears cannot be brushed aside; yet they must be balanced against the enormous good that is coming, and will certainly continue to come, from gene control technology.

Thalassemia, or Mediterranean anaemia, is a serious disorder of the blood. Haemolytic – blood-dissolving – is the appropriate medical adjective, since in this disorder the essence of blood, the red cells, are relentlessly destroyed and as a result the oxygen-carrying capacity of the blood is severely compromised. Enervating fatigue, physical weakness and lowered resistance to microbes are common. The child's bone marrow, the blood-forming organ, works overtime to try to re-supply red cells, but it is a futile effort that further weakens the child and compromises growth. Bones thin out and change shape, so the look of the child's face becomes abnormal, with enlargement of the head, protrusion of the upper teeth and lips, and broadening of the bridge of the nose.

The liver and spleen swell massively; heart failure is common. Doctors try to catch up with continual blood transfusions, but these have the side-effect of overloading the body with iron. Death due to lowered resistance, heart failure or iron overload occurs in the teens or, at best, in the twenties. I remember a young thalassemia patient in Boston whose constant hospital visits failed to relieve his pain. He turned to street drugs, almost in self-defence; it was the first time it occurred to me that drug abuse could be logical. He died of organ damage from iron overload, at twenty.

The disease begins with a genetic error, so it runs in families, and it is much more likely in populations where malaria is, or has been, prevalent – such as around the Mediterranean from which the disease takes its common name. Relatives of the victims, known as carriers, are partly resistant to malaria – the malaria-causing parasites, it turns out, need oxygen too and the compromised red cells of such people don't give them enough. What is a genetic advantage in combating malaria, however, can have tragic consequences when a child inherits the combined genes of two carriers. The incidence of thalassemia follows the worldwide distribution of malaria, for example, carriers make up fifteen to twenty per cent of the people of Vietnam and Cambodia. But even places where malaria is eradicated continue to have high rates of thalassemia; it is easier – and incidentally, less controversial – to outfox even a clever parasite than to alter the transmission of the genes.

Doctor Antonio Cao is planning to outfox the genes too. He lives and practises medicine in Sardinia, a beautiful Mediterranean island burdened with thalassemia – one in seven people is a carrier, and until 1974 around a hundred babies were born with the disease each year – one out of every 15 000 people in this population of one and a half million. Since malaria had been eliminated on the island by the early 1950s, there was no longer any advantage to being a carrier, and it is Doctor Cao's vision 'to overcome the problem of thalassemia in Sardinia'.

> As treatment became more effective we faced a huge health problem. The cost for each child was enormous. We didn't have enough blood donors and we didn't have enough money. If I hadn't established an effective prevention programme we would now have to treat an additional two thousand patients. This would be an impossible burden for this community.

Ironically, as doctors learned to use well-timed, frequent blood transfusions to prolong children's lives, their patients' very survival would have presented an insoluble problem. Even today Sardinia must import blood to care for the patients they have; yet there are now only four or five new patients born a year, out of many thousands of births, and these well cared for children live well beyond the limit of age ten that was typical two decades ago. In other words, Cao has come close to his original goal of eliminating thalassemia from Sardinia, while greatly enhancing the lives of its remaining victims.

He did this not with a medical instrument or a drug but with a public health programme and an institute of medical genetics, 'the largest and best organized in Italy'. As the architect of the programme and a leader of the institute – the Ospedale Regionale per le Micro-citemie – he has been able to combat the illness effectively. Television commercials urge Sardinians to donate blood, and while they are at it, to take a simple blood test that identifies carriers of thalassemia. Pregnant women carriers married to other carriers – around one in fifty couples – are urged to come in for a test at the institute at nine or ten weeks of pregnancy. One in four pregnancies of such couples will be a foetus destined not merely to be a carrier but to have the full-blown disorder. Couples notified of this sad fact usually choose abortion.

From a hundred down to five cases a year is an impressive achievement. But it raises certain questions. For one, to those who think abortion is murder, Doctor Cao's solution is no more acceptable than killing a thalassemia-stricken child would be. For another, it would seem to be difficult to draw the line. Doctor Cao's Ospedale tries to control not only thalassemia, but also both cystic fibrosis, a genetically caused lung disease, and muscular dystrophy in similar ways. He modelled his programme on efforts by Ashkenazic Jews in the US to eliminate their particular genetic burden: Tay-Sachs disease, a devastating form of mental retardation that always leads to death by the time the child has reached age two.

But where do we stop? Do we also consider aborting carriers of these defects? In the case of thalassemia, that would eliminate those most resistant to a possible reintroduction of malaria in the future. How about a disorder like Huntington's disease, a dreadful assault on the nervous system, but one that rarely starts before age thirty? How about the genetic form of Alzheimer's dementia, also dreadful, but emerging even later in life? How about susceptibilities, say to heart disease or breast cancer, that may or may not lead to diseases? And how about minor problems like a tendency to obesity or a need to wear glasses? How far will we carry our ability to eliminate defects, our zeal for human perfection?

There are those who believe we have already carried it far enough.

American critics within biology, such as Richard Lewontin and Jonathan Beckwith, both of Harvard University, have repeatedly sounded alarms about the dangers inherent in trying to improve human genetics. They point to the tragic history of this effort, called eugenics, especially in Germany under the Nazis. Forced sterilization of alleged mental defectives was only the mildest variety of their attempt to better the species. Legally sanctioned killing, not of foetuses but adults, was another step, and then the concept of defectives was extended to embrace all Jews and gypsies; killing elements of society labelled as biologically inferior, together with their children, would supposedly purify the European race.

This is a well-known story. What is less well known is that eugenic laws preceded the Nazis in Germany and that those laws in turn were modelled on American examples. Indiana became the first state to allow sterilization of the mentally ill as early as 1907. Two decades later twenty-eight other states had followed suit. Fifteen thousand individuals had been sterilized – 'unsexing' was another term – involuntarily by 1930. The attorney general of California, upholding its law, wrote: 'Degeneracy means that certain areas of brain cells or nerve centres of the individual are more highly or imperfectly developed than the other brain cells, and this causes an unstable state of the nerve system, which may manifest itself in insanity, criminality, idiocy, sexual perversion, or inebriety.' He went on to say that 'many of the confirmed inebriates, prostitutes, tramps, and criminals, as well as habitual paupers' belonged in this group eligible for legal castration.

Eugenic ideas became prominent in both Britain and the US. Eugenics had begun in Britain when Francis Galton coined the term in 1883. He was joined by Karl Pearson, a distinguished mathematician, and their ideas about improving the genetic stock of the British people were adopted and popularized by no less than H.G. Wells and George Bernard Shaw. Concerns about the genetic deterioration of the population through immigration and rapid breeding among the lower classes were widely discussed.

In the United States, however, the eugenic movement was far more consequential. Waiting periods between the application for a marriage licence and the wedding were imposed by law to give people time to reconsider genetically dubious matches. 'Fitter Families' contests – a strange amalgam of serious medical assessment and side-show – were held at state fairs in Kansas and elsewhere, with people being tested, measured and compared like livestock. IQ testing, developed during the First World War, began to be used mandatorily on prospective American immigrants, without such subtleties as ascertaining whether the subject spoke English, the language of the test. Leading American psychologists such as Lewis Terman and Robert Yerkes helped shape Congressional legislation that kept Jews, Italians and other eugenic 'undesirables' with 'low' IQs out. 'Science' reinforced previously existing racial and religious bigotry, and the resulting immigration quotas prevented hundreds of thousands, or possibly millions, of Jews in Nazi Europe from taking refuge in the United States.

In the pre-Nazi, democratic Germany of the Weimar republic, the spread of eugenic notions was also rapid. Two 'scientific' journals on 'racial hygiene' and 'social biology' had begun publication shortly after the turn of the century, and books on the subject were read and discussed widely by the end of the First World War. In 1920 a jurist and a psychiatrist, both well respected in Germany, published a book called *The Release and Destruction of Lives Devoid of Value*; it advocated not just sterilization, but large-scale euthanasia for the improvement of the race. In 1923 a director of health in Zwickau tried to persuade the Minister of the Interior that the time was right for eugenic sterilization. 'What we racial hygienists promote,' he wrote in a letter, 'is not at all new or unheard of. In a cultured nation of the first order, the United States of America, that which we strive toward was introduced and tested long ago.' The sceptical minister ordered a study, and was convinced by the resulting report; if America could do it, so could Germany. A decade later, after Hitler came to power, the 'lives devoid of value' began to number in the millions. A decade after that, those millions were actually being destroyed.

Every step in this process was viewed as stemming from and consistent with advances in medical science – 'racial hygiene'. Sober scientific institutes, weighty treatises and technical journals all promoted race purification as a public health measure. It was not a coincidence that at the Auschwitz death camp a physician selected the small number of people in each trainload whom they considered fit enough to live and engage in slave labour or forced prostitution for a time. The remaining majority had to be officially, medically certified as suitable for the gas chambers; each consignment of victims required a document that carried the signature of a physician.

So in addition to the universal human soul-searching inspired by these facts, medicine must undergo its own particular search. We must ask, not just, How could these things have happened? but also How could medicine have become so perverted as to play such a central role? And, of course, we must ask whether medicine could be so perverted again.

For Baptist fundamentalists, Jehovah's Witnesses and some others, the answer is that it is happening right now in all countries where abortion is routine. These are the kinds of people who compare Etienne-Emile Baulieu to Hitler, and who see routine abortion as mass murder. These people are in a small minority, much smaller than the 'pro-life' contingent, and even they are not consistent in their beliefs; for example, they don't mourn when they have a late menstrual period, which is often a very early spontaneous abortion.

But one does not need to be an extremist to see some analogy with Nazi 'eugenics' when abortion is specifically used to eliminate defectives – lives, one might say, devoid of value. Not surprisingly perhaps, some of the most sensitive monitoring of this unsettling possibility is occurring today in Germany, where the experience of carrying and bearing a child has become intensively medicalized. As in the US, German obstetricians have been sued for 'wrongful life' by women who have borne abnormal babies and have felt that the doctor should have warned them so that they could have chosen abortion. One British obstetrician whose patient had a Downs syndrome child – this form of mental retardation is easily detected at ten weeks of pregnancy – was ordered by the court to pay a large sum in damages because, mistakenly thinking the mother was thirty-seven (the cut-off age for testing being thirty-eight), he had failed to recommend testing.

With precedents like this, obstetricians everywhere are growing edgy about allowing an abnormal pregnancy to continue. They monitor pregnancies closely and strongly urge their patients to undergo prenatal testing. Yet not all women respond well to so much technology. Just as in the 1970s women in many countries began to insist on increasingly natural childbirth, and got it, today in Germany a similar resistance is emerging in response to prenatal testing. In Bremen an organization called CARA is a shop-front counselling centre begun by women who are all health professionals, and provides pregnant women with advice on an alternative to the usual medicalized experience. And Bremen's disabled women's group urges that disability be viewed as part of the normal variety of life.

Anne Waldschmidt, disabled from birth by a rare genetic disease, deeply fears the tyranny of perfect health: 'Medicine reflects our culture, and in a high technology society we have become concerned with perfection. As we strive for this perfection we seem to be less and less tolerant of imperfection. We are never going to wipe out birth defects, and technology is changing the experience of pregnancy.'

Since she has been an advisor on genetic engineering and reproductive technologies to the influential Green Party, her words may some day alter policy. She says unequivocally: 'Society should accept such things as thalassemia – otherwise where do you stop?' Prenatal selection is seen by her as a more subtle continuation of the eugenic tradition of Germany's Nazi past. Health, as Waldschmidt puts it, can become 'a totalitarian concept'.

It is both moving and persuasive to see Germans trying to draw a clear line in the shifting eugenic sand. And those who view their fears as greatly overblown might consider recent events in China. Several provinces – Fujian, Guangdong, Hena, Liaoning and Sichuan, with a combined population of 320 million – have promulgated compulsory sterilization laws, and a national eugenics law has been under discussion for several years. Trends in China today are eerily similar to the popular spread and legal sanctioning of eugenics in the US, Britain and Europe during the early to mid-twentieth century. In Gansu, in the north-west, and Liaoning, in the north-east, for example, certain categories of individuals have to undergo examinations before they are given permission to marry. If viewed as unfit, they are barred from marrying pending sterilization, and if they elude sterilization and begin a pregnancy, they can be required to have an abortion.

People subject to these laws include those with mental illnesses, mental retardation and hereditary diseases. Sterilization is invoked if both potential spouses are retarded 'at middle degree' or if one is retarded 'at severe degree'. If these laws are emulated at the national level – a step supported by many health officials and by the Chinese Association for the Handicapped – approximately fifty million physically or mentally handicapped people throughout China could be affected. Although an estimated twenty million of these people may actually have hereditary diseases, the majority acquired their handicaps because of environmental factors and sterilization is therefore anyway pointless for them. But even if retardation is not necessarily hereditary, it is thought to be so in China.

Western scientists are agreed that the Chinese programme is an extremely crude one, in addition to being unjust, but Chinese intellectuals who defend it cite the ancient Confucian tradition that subordinates the individual to the good of society. They as well as health officials readily resort to language such as that used by Zhang Zhongjian, chief of the women and children's office in Liaoning province's health department: 'The purpose of making the law and regulations is to raise the population quality and reduce the state's burden and family misfortunes'; or that of the national health minister Chen Minzhang, who told a 1990 conference that the low quality of the population has become a 'heavy millstone around our neck in the journey to catch up with international competition and modernize'.

Clearly what is intended here is not very far from 'racial hygiene'. Thousands of compulsory sterilizations and an unknown number of mandatory abortions had already taken place within a year of the first law's enactment in Gansu province in November 1988. In time, if the national law is enacted, millions will be affected. As if to close the circle of similarity to the Nazi past, foreign critics have warned that these laws may be invoked especially against China's ethnic minorities in impoverished rural areas. Such minorities, who have received at best questionable treatment from the Chinese in the past, include Tibetans, Mongols and Turkic minorities in Gansu province, as well as Koreans in Liaoning.

And another oppressed group that is not a minority – females – is also the target of selective abortion. This has happened not only in China, where the push for the one-child family has made having a son the first time all the more urgent, but even more so in some northern provinces of India, where prenatal diagnosis has been used surreptitiously for the sole purpose of determining sex, and virtually all girls are aborted in some samples of tested foetuses. These are parts of India where extreme preference for males is deeply embedded in the culture. But even in Britain and the States, physicians providing prenatal diagnosis are uneasy at times that they are actually serving the goals of some parents who absolutely insist on having boys, or, occasionally, girls.

Meanwhile, in those same Western countries, the most costly and the most broadly organized initiative in the history of biomedical research has captured – or captivated – many of the most talented minds who ever applied science to human welfare. James Watson, Walter Gilbert, and Leroy Hood, are only a few of the stellar scientists who have made leadership in this new programme their top research priority. Their enthusiasm has spread to thousands of younger scientists, and to science funding administrators, who have made this programme the closest thing in biology to 'Big Science' – the blue-chip physics of massive particle accelerators and space stations.

The programme in question is the Human Genome Project, and its goal is to identify and determine the chemical sequences of all the 100 000 or so genes that make each of us what we are, at least biologically. Many of those genes are being pursued individually – personally, one might almost say – by scientists who realize that they hold the keys to some of the tightest locks in the whole realm of human disease. An example is the gene for sickle-cell anaemia, a much more severe cousin of thalassemia, but one that overwhelmingly affects blacks – with pain that can make victims wish for death; or the gene for cystic fibrosis, the most widespread genetic syndrome affecting whites, in which sticky lung secretions gradually choke the life out of the young victim; or the critical genes that switch on or stifle the runaway cell growth that creates cancer.

But in parallel with this specific gene-hunting, which understandably grabs headlines, the unsung common soldiers of the Human Genome Project slog away month after month decoding the whole, almost endless string of highly structured DNA that is triply coiled upon itself in the nucleus of every human cell. (Gilbert invites us to think of it as the information contained in a thousand, thousand-page telephone books.) Along the way, in this tedious but necessary task, they will pick up on numerous genes whose existence we now do not even suspect, suggesting new and possibly easy paths in biomedical science. A few of these discoveries will no doubt produce a table-slapping 'aha!' reaction when a new, unexpected gene is matched to an old and baffling disease. But for the most part the effort will slowly but surely unravel the code, molecule by molecule and ultimately gene by gene.

The project is meant to be completed within two decades, but its reverberations will echo in medicine for many decades more. And their impact will certainly not be limited to such crude procedures as prenatal diagnosis followed by abortion. Through an elegant process called 'reverse genetics', sequenced genes are being followed through to the proteins they generate; where these are deficient or abnormal they will be augmented or replaced. Protein functions that become apparent through this process will lead to new paths in rational drug design, and many new, effective drugs will then be found by following through on these genetic insights with old-fashioned pharmaceutical methods. Such secrets will be unlocked as how to make replacement skin for people with severe burns and how to orchestrate reconnections in the severed spinal cord of a paraplegic – secrets that will start with genetic research but that in the application will have nothing directly to do with genes. Yet genes themselves will be delivered into patients – they already have been in limited ways, using carefully modified viruses as vehicles – and these genes will correct or replace defective ones in the owner's original collection.

And for those for whom abortion is not an option, but who want to abolish, say, muscular dystrophy from their families for ever, it will one day be possible to subject their fertilized eggs to 'gene surgery'. Such correction of a sequence in a gene, right in the fertilized egg, will decisively negate the harsh reality of the defect, which had stood as truth for perhaps hundreds of generations. What was a burden and an anguish during century after century will become a mere memory.

But we will still have to sort out just what is being eliminated. Those who believe we need to accept genetically caused physical handicaps as a natural part of the richness and variety of human life will probably always be a small minority. Even if we agree with the main thrust of their argument, there will always and everywhere be environmental damage; acquired illnesses, chemical exposures, accidents and violence will produce enough handicapped people – they, not patients with genetic flaws, make up most of the disabled today – to satisfy any philosopher's need for human variety. Looking back on the history of the conquest of disease, we find some people decrying the effort to cure syphilis on the grounds that such a cure would foster immorality; or obliquely admiring tuberculosis because it appeared to be associated with aesthetic sensitivity. Perhaps we should not cure leprosy, because what sort of phony world would it be without lepers? There is no reason to single out genetic disorders when assessing the philosophical value of imperfection; and conversely, if it is well to abolish acquired disability, it should also be well to abolish the genetic kind.

But the questions about where to draw the line in the quest for perfection will remain, and no more strikingly than in the realm of behaviour and intelligence, where passions run high in response to human variety, and where the greatest difficulties are encountered in defining disability. To take an example, the elimination of Down's syndrome foetuses following prenatal chromosomal diagnosis for women in their late thirties or older has become routine in a number of Western countries. Yet even though this syndrome produces mental retardation, some affected children function at quite a high level; moreover, the human value of such children to their families, friends and schoolmates, not to mention themselves, is not scientifically definable. The issue is partly moot, since many babies with the syndrome will continue to be born to younger women who aren't routinely tested; but the serious philosophical questions remain.

A different sort of question is raised by Huntington's disease, a devastating form of brain degeneration, but one that begins only in the thirties or forties. It destroyed the popular folk-singer Woody Guthrie, but not before allowing him a rich and full creative life. In some cases the first symptoms appear as psychiatric ones, so the syndrome proves the power of a simple genetic defect decisively to alter the human mind. The disease was also the first in which a human gene of any kind was linked to a part of a chromosome, using the new methods of molecular genetics. Within a few years of the genetic defect being located, scientists offered a diagnostic test. People who had lost a parent to the disease had long known that they had a fifty-fifty chance of developing it themselves. Now they could find out, yes or no, could plan for shorter lives, or for their deaths. Theoretically, the diagnosis should soon be available prenatally; and many people in affected families will then no doubt exercise their right to abort such a foetus. But would we really have wanted Woody Guthrie not to have been born?

For Alzheimer's disease, the most widespread form of senility coming late in life, the parallel questions are even more nagging. There are genetic forms of the Alzheimer's type of senility, running in families, and as with Huntington's disease, we may want to know in advance if we are headed for Alzheimer's. Few things are feared more by older people today than having a wise old age turned into a helpless second infancy; in which they are robbed of memory itself, and thus of most meaning to life. But are we going to abort a foetus because it may become a demented old man or woman after seventy years of normal life? Indeed, are we going to abort the majority of foetuses, since the greater the age we live, the more likely it is that we will eventually get the disease.

In contrast to Huntington's disease, much is known about how Alzheimer's works. The affected brain has certain distinctive features under the microscope – plaques and tangles, they are called – and brain chemists have begun to figure out what those tiny but decisive abnormalities are made of. One defective protein found in the tangles, beta-amyloid, is apparently made from a gene on chromosome 21. There are more details emerging, and year by year, experiment by experiment, scientists are slowly moving towards the goal of a complete understanding of this tragic illness, from the biochemical defect in the gene (not yet known), through the abnormal protein or proteins, to the changes in brain structure, to the loss of memory and self-control. Every step of this path will offer opportunities for thwarting the process of Alzheimer's – using as yet undiscovered drugs – once the path is properly traced and the process understood. Genetics will be perhaps the most crucial research tool, but the treatment may be conventional and far removed from the actual genes.

Still another genetic brain disorder, PKU or phenylketonuria, begins its assault on the human mind within hours of birth. It is clearly controlled by the genes, yet it has been solved for a long time, long before any details of the location or structure of the gene were known. How this was done is an object lesson in the surprising solutions we can expect for genetic disorders. The disease got its name because of phenylketones, chemical products found in the victim's urine. Old-fashioned biochemistry had shown, long before the era of modern genetics, that these ketones came from excessive amounts of phenylalanine, an ordinary amino acid not only present in most proteins but also essential in human diet.

Elementary chemical reasoning led to the conclusion that victims of this genetic disease lacked a crucial enzyme – one of the large helper-molecules that speeds up the body's normal reactions and helps convert the phenylalanine into certain neurotransmitters, hormones and other products. Without it, some of those products can be made in other ways, but the phenylalanine eaten normally every day piles up in the brain until it begins to poison brain cells, resulting in severe mental retardation.

The physicians of the day did not wait for the genetic revolution to repair or exclude the defective gene, but attacked the disease on a completely different front: they changed the diet. The result was successful prevention of the disease, merely by giving the child a specially prepared diet without any phenylalanine. A genetic disease was thus basically cured by a method that not only had nothing to do with genes, but also nothing to do with eugenics. The genes were simply left in the population, and instead of trying to change them, the environment was changed. This is a perfect demonstration of the interaction between genes and environment, of the simple fact that defective genes are only defective in relation to some environment; if you change that environment it may become meaningless to think of the gene as defective.

Similarly, by supplying corrective lenses we render the genetic 'defect' causing myopia powerless; with countless work-saving machines we abolish the ancient evolutionary superiority of muscular power. Thus the genes for near-sightedness and relative muscular weakness must inevitably become more common in the human population. We don't worry about these common genetic 'defects' and about the eugenic consequences of their spread for the human species, because we know that they have ceased to matter in the environments that we humans create for ourselves; that, in a real sense, they are no longer defects at all.

Philosophical doubts have been raised about the goal of eliminating even severe genetic defects, and cautious policy questions must be raised about any attempt to eliminate mild ones – characteristics which some doctors see as defects, but which most others see as part of normal human variation. But few enthusiasts of molecular genetics have confronted an even more distressing possibility: that in their zeal to eliminate variations that look like defects, they may inadvertently destroy variations that are advantageous. This possibility clearly exists in the case of manic depressive illness.

Also known as bipolar mood disorder, this serious psychiatric problem carries patients through enormous mood swings, from manias characterized by a fast-talking flight of half-baked ideas and danger-ously risky behaviour to depressions marked by inactivity, helplessness, hopelessness and a seemingly inescapable sadness. 'My mind's not right,' wrote the American poet Robert Lowell, who suffered from the illness. 'I hear/My spirit sob in each blood cell,/As if my hand were at its throat .../I myself am hell.' Before the advent of lithium and other treatments discovered by modern psychiatry, the illness often ended in death by the victim's own hand.

It is clearly a disorder, if any psychiatric entity is. And it clearly has an inherited component. Studies of twins, at least one of whom has manic depressive illness, have shown that if the other twin is genetically identical, he or she has between a sixty-seven and eighty per cent likelihood of also becoming a manic depressive. But the corresponding percentages for non-identical twins are far lower. Similarly, people who were adopted in infancy and who later commit suicide have *biological* relatives with a suicide rate six- to twelve-fold higher than their *adoptive* relatives, or than either the biological or adoptive relatives of non-suicidal adoptees. According to Doctor Elliot Gershon, a leading authority on psychiatric genetics, the chance of a person with manic depressive illness having a child who will grow up to have either the same illness or very serious depressions is roughly one in four. It is of course arguable how far environmental factors need to be taken into account in this or similar illnesses, but a major contribution from the genes is beyond question.

One attempt to use molecular genetics to link the gene for manic depressive illness to a particular chromosome proved to be a false start. Data on a large extended family among the Amish of Pennsylvania, where there were a number of cases of the disorder, seemed to link the defect to a genetic marker on chromosome 11. But this link dissolved when two family members who lacked the marker later developed the illness. Another series of studies linking it to the X chromosome – near the gene for colour blindness – is probably more reliable, but also probably only accounts for a subset of manic depressives. Yet even in this preliminary state of research, patients come to Doctor Gershon with requests for definitive prenatal tests that will enable them to abort foetuses destined to have the illness.

He routinely discourages them, not only because of the vague state of present knowledge, but also because these illnesses are now largely treatable.

False starts and continuing puzzles aside, science may well get a genetic handle on some forms of this disorder, comparable to the one it has on, say, Huntington's disease, within another decade or so. Some doctors, and certainly some patients, will undoubtedly be tempted to use prenatal testing and selective abortion to stave off the disease in future children. But they will have to come to grips with another set of facts, now at least equally scientific: we may not know what genetic markers manic depressive illness is linked to, but we know for sure that it is often linked to creativity.

This is scarcely a new idea; Aristotle no doubt exaggerated when he wrote that 'all extraordinary men distinguished in philosophy, politics, poetry and the arts are evidently melancholic'. But the personal histories of Beethoven, Dickens, Van Gogh and Newton, among many other creative geniuses, bear him out. It was only in the late 1980s and early 1990s, however, that the connection between mood disorders and creativity was scientifically established. We can now say that although most creative people are not mentally ill, and although most people with mood disorders are not especially creative, these two forms of human experience occur together more often than can be explained by chance alone.

Kay Jamison, a psychologist at the John Hopkins Hospital who is an authority on manic depression, studied forty-seven eminent British writers and artists. Each had been awarded one or more of the top British prizes in their field, for example, the London *Evening Standard* Drama Award, or the Queen's Gold Medal for Poetry, or had comparable other recognition. Thirty-eight per cent of these enormously accomplished people had been treated for mood disorders, three-fourths with medication or even hospitalization. In addition, thirty per cent more had experienced what they described as severe mood swings. The first figure compares with an estimated five or six per cent for the population at large.

Psychiatrist Nancy Andreasen was a literary scholar before entering medicine, and she later decided to study writers. Thirty faculty members at the renowned University of Iowa Writers' Workshop were compared with thirty other professionals matched for age, sex and education. Twenty-four of the writers (eighty per cent) had experienced some sort of mood disorder, as opposed to nine (thirty per cent) of the control group. Thirteen of the writers had had manic depressive illness in some measure, which was true of only three of the controls. During the fifteen years of the study, two of the thirty writers took their own lives.

Doctor Hagop Akiskal, a psychiatrist at the University of Tennessee, and his wife and associate Kareen Akiskal, a Parisian art dealer, studied painters, sculptors and writers in France and blues musicians in the American south-east. While they found no evidence of the more severe forms of manic depressive illness in these groups, they did find definite evidence of marked mood swings – more moderate mood disorders. And in a separate study they did of 750 American psychiatric patients, this link was strongly confirmed in the other direction: people with moderate mood disorders are more likely to have significant, recognized creative ability.

Finally, Ruth Richards, a psychologist at the Harvard Medical School, has found creativity to be over-represented not only among patients with severe or moderate manic depressive cycles, but also among their relatives, as compared to the relatives of 'normal' controls. Richards and her colleagues proposed that the genes for manic depressive illness are like the genes for thalassemia and sickle-cell anaemia in one important respect. The people who have high doses of them may be maladapted, but those who are only 'carriers' may have a distinct advantage. In the case of the genetic anaemias, carrier-relatives are more resistant to malaria (although this is no advantage in the absence of malarial parasites). In the case of manic depressive illness, relatives are apparently more creative.

It is difficult to conceive of a human environment in which superior creativity is not an advantage, and the roster of people with serious mood disorders includes some of the most revered creators in the past – Blake, Coleridge, Balzac, Goethe, Handel and Tchaikovsky, to name a few; not to mention leaders such as Winston Churchill and Abraham Lincoln, who suffered from quite serious mood swings. If we find genes responsible for the manic depressive type of psychiatric illness and set out systematically to eliminate them, we will in all likelihood also eliminate some of the potential for creativity that in the past has given us so much that we would not want to lose.

This caution should be borne in mind when considering the strange case of Tourette's syndrome, which is currently the focus of a wave of intense interest in the small but growing circle of scientists and physicians who study it. Named after the French physician who first described it in 1885, Tourette's until a few years ago was a little known medical curiosity. Most doctors who recognized the name would have told you a fascinating tale of rare patients with uncontrollable tics, not only muscular but verbal ones, with the patient often repeatedly shouting embarassingly vulgar words in public settings, unable to stop themselves. A few doctors might also have known that Tourette's could often be treated with haloperidol, a drug that blocks the receptors for dopamine, one of the brain's internal transmitter chemicals, much the way RU 486 blocks the receptors for the hormone progesterone.

But over the last five or six years there has been a dramatic change in thinking about Tourette's syndrome. What was once seen as a rare disorder now seems, in varied and subtle forms, a relatively common one. What was once a mystery in terms of cause and effect has been replaced by a partial explanation: genes play an important role. And what was once a little backwater in the byways of specialized neurology has become almost a thoroughfare, not only for sober medical study but for questionable philosophical speculation.

Groups of researchers at Yale, at the University of Rochester and at the City of Hope Hospital in Los Angeles have become fascinated by Tourette's, and in following patients with the problem have made some important discoveries. Under the leadership of Doctor Roger Kurlan, investigators at Rochester and Yale followed a clue presented in 1983 by a Tourette's patient, David Janzen, who was very worried by a misdiagnosis – he had been told he had Huntington's disease – and very eager to help when he found out it was Tourette's. Fortunately for science, he came from a large family of Mennonites in a tiny town in rural Alberta, Canada. His many relatives in the pacifist Christian sect were local, easy to trace and for the most part cooperative; 159 were personally interviewed.

The result was much new information about the disorder. For one thing, most of the fifty-four family members diagnosed with some form of the syndrome – over eighty per cent – were never bothered enough by their symptoms to seek medical help; contrary to received wisdom, their Tourette's was usually very mild. David Janzen himself had disturbing repetitive outbursts of movements and words, but his affected cousins tended to have only a tic or two, perhaps a noticeable but untroublesome facial twitch.

Doctor David Pauls, a Yale colleague of Kurlan's, explored a more diverse set of smaller families related to Tourette's syndrome patients in Connecticut. In addition to tics, which affected mostly male relatives, ten per cent of the family members suffered from out of the ordinary obsessive thoughts or compulsive acts, for example, having to get dressed over and over again for hours each morning. These people were mostly women. Pauls began to think that perhaps the same genetic background could be expressed in some relatives (mainly boys and men) as tics or full-blown Tourette's syndrome, while in others (mainly girls and women) the same gene or genes produced more complex obsessions or compulsions, less tied to bursts of muscle activity. Pauls and his colleague James Leckman found it hard to interpret the pattern of heredity of Tourette's by sticking to the core symptoms, but if the relatives with obsessive-compulsive disorders were included, a clear inheritance pattern emerged.

Meanwhile Doctor David Comings, a geneticist at the City of Hope Hospital, became convinced of a quite different genetic pattern, showing the large degree of uncertainty on this small frontier of medicine. Yet Comings was willing to go much further, not only in his scientific interpretations but in his approach to patients and their families:

> It's often been felt that there are separate genes for alcoholism, for schizophrenia, for depression, for Tourette's syndrome, for attention deficit disorder. One of the things we seem to be finding is that there is a similar set of genes that are at the basis of a lot of these different disorders . . .
>
> One could argue that up to ten to twenty per cent of the population has some type of genetic behavioural problem . . . All you have to do is look at the problems with alcoholism, the problems with depression, the problem with manic depressive disorder, to see that they have an extraordinarily severe impingement on the functioning of society, and if we can begin to make some dent in this and understand it and treat these conditions – especially identify them early in life and get the children treated before they have these breakdowns or problems – I think it would be an enormous benefit to society.

In this speech all the worst fears of those who cite the abuses of eugenics are realized. Doctor Comings, who is not a psychiatrist, deems up to twenty per cent of the human population to be abnormal in some way in their behaviour. He would use genetic medicine to lop off twenty per cent of the variety in human action, personality, mood – in effect, twenty per cent of the human spirit. Excessive activity, drinking, antisocial behaviour, sadness, all these and more would be subject to correction in his vision of future medicine. For his present patients, he uses clonidine, primarily a blood-pressure medication, to treat not just tics or Tourette's syndrome, but many of these other problems as well. If any of the behaviours change, he considers the drug a success.

Soberer minds bristle at this confident, all-inclusive approach. Doctor Kenneth Kidd, a leading psychiatric geneticist who works with Pauls at Yale, says, 'I think that the case is definitely not proven for this very broad involvement of a single gene that causes Tourette's and many other disorders. Our own data collected here at Yale very strongly argued the other way.' He also says, in a tone of concern, that 'people with Tourette's syndrome are starting to call up and say, "I want my children tested for this gene." There is a lot of misunderstanding out there.'

Of course, unlike the case for thalassemia, Huntington's disease or PKU, there is no test for Tourette's syndrome, genetic or otherwise. Yet incautious statements to the media continue to raise false hopes and fears. Sue Levi-Pearl, head of the Tourette's Syndrome Association in the States, is worried that 'folks with Tourette's syndrome are getting information – for instance, that their disorder is distinctly related to alcoholism, to addiction, sexual aberration – and so they become very, very frightened ... A woman called and said that her daughter has a brother with Tourette's and that she was pregnant and now she was not only concerned about having a baby perhaps with Tourette's syndrome but that this baby would also be an alcoholic. Now that's utterly absurd. There are too many questions that have yet to be answered.'

As for treatment, Doctor Comings places his confidence in clonidine, delivered through a patch on the skin, but other authorities on the disorder, such as Arthur and Elaine Shapiro, believe that 'clonidine is only rarely effective', and point to the large number of patients who get better spontaneously and to the lack of proper drug studies. Even haloperidol, a more standard and probably better treatment for Tourette's, has yet to be proved effective in a well-planned controlled trial. Both these drugs can have serious side-effects, and although each is approved for other purposes, the balance of risks and benefits for Tourette's is far from clear.

Doctor Donald Cohen, a psychiatrist at Yale, also uses clonidine, but only in the context of a much more complex and varied treatment. He believes that 'the best people to be involved are people who can see the child as a whole person, realize what he's experiencing and have a view of where he's going to be developing. And that wouldn't be someone who's just interested in the tics and getting rid of the tics.' Tommy is a young man who has been one of his patients since childhood. He is self-possessed, articulate and sensitive as he describes his difficult childhood, when he was often ostracized because of his tics. Yet he feels less angry at his thoughtless childhood friends than his mother does on his behalf. 'His philosophy,' she says, 'is "Well mother, what can you expect? ... they're not taught to be understanding ... and so it's not their fault." I remember him going out and saying "Look, I have a problem but I'm not a problem. I do things that seem crazy but I'm not crazy." '

Tommy himself says wisely, 'And now that I'm older and I'm just like everybody else – quote unquote "everybody else", whatever that means – I deal with problems a lot better than most other people because the problems I have now to me are very minor. It's just another thing to deal with.' His mother later underscores his specialness, obviously in part gained from his triumph over his illness: 'We would never turn the clock back and we would never give Tommy back ever, because he's just a wonderful human being, he's kind and caring and affectionate ... he's a gift to us.' Yet even she concedes that if she had the choice in the future, she would be tempted to avoid what she knows from experience would be 'a terrible, terrible struggle'.

In Sydney, Australia, Elizabeth and Andrew Hearne are soon to have their second child. Through prenatal testing, they have become well acquainted with the baby, for a very simple reason: they do not want a child with muscular dystrophy. Elizabeth – Libby – had watched her brother Greg deteriorate slowly throughout his childhood and then die at the age of eighteen. They know that even today there is no treatment. Five years earlier she had seen her sister Christine give birth to a son with the ailment; he too would probably be in a wheelchair by his teens and might not live past twenty. Christine had had a blood test just two years before prenatal testing was possible, and the test had been falsely reassuring. Her son Nicholas had been the one child in fifty born with muscular dystrophy after such a favourable blood test result. Libby had had CVS – chorionic villus sampling – a newer, more complex and more advanced test that takes cells from the placenta around the tenth week of pregnancy. She and Andrew felt strongly against bringing another child with muscular dystrophy into the world: 'We'd lived with it once, and for it to happen again, and Greg was still alive when Christine had Nicholas. It just ... it just seemed so unfair for it to happen twice in a family.'

The test had been reassuring, but the baby was a boy, and since it is usually only boys who get this type of muscular dystrophy – called Duchenne's, it comes from a gene on the X chromosome – they had remained uneasy. The family had already had one experience of false reassurance. With a girl Libby would have felt sure, even though – like her first child, her daughter Alex – she could be a carrier: 'That could be a problem in later life, but hopefully in twenty years time they'll have ... she won't have to go through any of this at all.'

Libby has high hopes for the genetic revolution, and for medical science in general. But in the real world of today, she says, 'We're doing as much as possible, as much as can be done at the moment, to try and ensure that we have a healthy child ... It's just not fair on the child ... it's not fair on Alex ... it's not fair on us and all our family to –' But she breaks off here to say something different: 'It's horrible to think you can be so choosy ... like you can say, Oh that baby is not good enough for me, or there is something wrong with it, so it's not good enough.' Her husband Andrew comes in to say, 'But nature does that anyway.' Libby knows, but she is still not quite comfortable with the power genetic medicine has given her.

Clearly these are not the sort of people who would abuse the privilege of genetic diagnosis. The Hearnes gave birth to a perfect baby boy – or rather, to a boy with only the garden-variety imperfections that all babies have. Their happiness was great indeed.

Anne Waldschmidt, the disabled woman in Bremen who fears the intolerance of imperfection, is right when she says we will never eliminate birth defects. But if we can take Doctor Anthony Cao's success in Sardinia in reducing thalassemia births by ninety-five per cent, and repeat that success with sickle-cell anaemia and cystic fibrosis, with muscular dystrophy and Tay-Sachs disease, and with other unequivocally tragic genetic syndromes – with these efforts alone we will have received our money's worth from the genetic revolution, even if it were not expected to help cure AIDS and cancer. Yet Waldschmidt's fears are being realized in China, even as Western doctors decry those fears as implausible. When the line is crossed between birth control and forced sterilization, from a woman's right to choose to compulsory abortion, then we may indeed be on the slippery slope that runs down to Auschwitz.

But as for voluntary choice of genetic counselling, selective fertilization, prenatal testing and abortion, who has the right to stand between a family and those options? Since the family will bear the brunt of the impact of disability, it would seem that the family has the right to take any available medical measures to avoid that impact. These measures will be ever more varied and powerful. But surely a vigilant society with full respect for civil rights can continue to tell the difference between the removal of a foetus destined for a short, painful life and the kind of 'eugenic' nightmare finally realized by the Nazis. And eventually selective fertilization, or even 'gene surgery', may make such programmes as Doctor Cao's workable *without* having to use abortion.

But we must recognize how large a set of questions we are facing. Of the three billion molecular beads that are strung together to make up the human DNA, probably millions are polymorphic – normally differing from one individual to the next. Each of us carries five or six mutations – genes that are clearly defective in one of the two copies we carry; genes that, if paired with another matched defective one in the complex dance of mating, would produce a devastating illness. We cannot go after all these defects, and we would never want, I hope, to go after the normal variation.

Lewis Thomas, the famed physician-essayist, has written, 'The capacity to blunder slightly is the real marvel of DNA. Without this special attribute, we would still be anaerobic bacteria and there would be no music ... it is no accident at all that mutations occur; the molecule of DNA was ordained from the beginning to make small mistakes.' What he means is that without damage to genes there would be no variation, and without variation there would not only be no evolution, there would be no unpredictable variety in the world of the sort that makes life worth living. The problem is to find some way of defining a 'slight' blunder that makes it possible to differentiate it from a colossal one. This, it turns out, will not be easy. If we agree that families have a right to select away major disabilities like muscular dystrophy, on what grounds can families be discouraged from selecting away manic depressive illness, with its connection to creativity? Or, for that matter, do we even have a right to discourage people from using the new technology merely to select for a certain sex?

Yet it is not a 'brave new world' of total control that genetic medicine seeks, but the same goal that has inspired physicians since ages before Hippocrates: the rational conquest of illness and the reduction – rational or otherwise – of human suffering. There are huge philosophical questions, yes, and these should be raised again and again, but still we should have the confidence to go forward.

CHAPTER 5

RANDOM CUTS

At a recent physicians' dinner I attended, a joke was told by one doctor on another, in the course of honouring him near the end of a long career. 'I was talking with Doctor Randall the other day,' he said, 'and chanced to ask him how he would change his life if he should win the Florida lottery. He looked thoughtful for a while. Since the lottery was then going to pay about forty million dollars, he had a lot to think about. "Well," he finally said. "I suppose I would continue to operate. But I would only do indicated procedures."'

Indicated is doctor-talk for justified, purposeful, needed. The joke was revealing. Every physician in the room who had ever performed an operation, ordered a CAT scan or hospitalized a patient without feeling sure that the step was really necessary and in the patient's best interest, rather than in the interest, say, of defensive medicine, scientific curiosity or profit – and that meant almost everyone present – must have felt the bite of that jibe. All the doctors laughed with as well as at Doctor Randall.

But of course they were also laughing at their patients. It is an impressive irony that in the American system, where tens of millions of uninsured or under-insured people are denied needed procedures, many millions of others *able* to pay are subjected to needless ones. However, this practice follows long medical tradition on both sides of the Atlantic. In some places in the ancient world, the sick had holes drilled in their skulls to let out damaging spirits, and for most of European history blood-letting was a standard medical response to a wide variety of illnesses.

These procedures were done in good faith – not just with the goal of collecting a fee. The doctors and patients involved believed that they worked; they felt that they had to do something, and these procedures were the best they had to offer. Because the beliefs were strong, the psychological impact of the procedures was strong as well; and through the placebo effect, they may have produced improvement. But there was never any evidence that they worked for the reasons doctors did them, or that they achieved the goals they were done for beyond the placebo effect. Yet few doctors or patients at the time had the slightest doubt that they were the right thing to do.

In recent times, under the same broad umbrella of medical self-assurance, there was a fashion for tonsillectomies. In 1934 a study done in New York City revealed that of 1000 eleven-year-olds in the state schools, 611 had had their tonsils removed. The other 389 were evaluated by a panel of physicians for possible tonsillectomies and the operation was recommended for 174 more. (Fortunately, these children were not actually sent to surgery!) Different physicians looked at the remaining 215 and chose to 'operate' on 99 more, leaving only 116 from the original 1000 'surgery-free'. These 116 were evaluated by a third panel of doctors, who recommended 51 more of them for surgery.

This pattern is stunning. Second opinions are usually thought of as a way to *reduce* the likelihood of surgery, but in this group of a thousand schoolchildren, ninety-three per cent of them had, or were recommended to have, surgery when up to three opinions were given. Today tonsillectomies are done on only a small fraction of children, but a decades-long surgical fad swept millions of British and American children up in its over-enthusiasm. As one of those millions, I remember waking from anaesthesia crying and spitting blood, surrounded by other children in the consulting-room assembly-line, all doing likewise. I was five, and the year was 1951 – right in the midst of the enormous enthusiasm for tonsillectomies.

What happened subsequently should be a lesson in humility for all surgeons, in fact for all physicians. Doctor John Wennberg and his colleagues at the Harvard School of Public Health studied the rates of tonsil removal in thirteen Vermont hospital service areas beginning in 1969. In that year the rate for the US as a whole was comparable to the Vermont rate. Yet there was a *thirteen-fold* difference between the highest- and lowest-rate hospital districts in the state. These facts were reported back to Vermont doctors through the state medical society, and tonsillectomies in Vermont began to decline at a rate that far exceeded the national decline that began around the same time – the fad was then ending. By 1973 the Vermont rate was forty-six per cent below what it had been in 1969, and was also far lower than the national rate.

Furthermore, this pattern of decline was greatest by far in the hospital district that had had the highest rate at the outset. Here, the drop was eighty-nine per cent in five years, from being more than triple the national rate in 1969 to less than half the national rate in 1973, and this despite a forty-six per cent national decline in the same period. Careful analysis led Wennberg and his colleagues to credit the district's sharp drop mainly to feedback – simply letting the doctors know where they stood in relation to other doctors.

Writing in 1977, the authors said that 'at least for a decade there has been a decline in the popularity of tonsillectomies in the United States' and they attributed much of this to review of the procedures done and feedback of the information to practising doctors. This was good news, though describing tonsillectomies in terms of their 'popularity' seems disconcertingly like discussing the ups and downs of television sitcoms or rock music groups.

A similar fad had come and gone in Canada, England and Wales, and the decline in tonsillectomies in Britain from 1970 to 1976 (thirty-five per cent) was even greater than that in the States (twenty-three per cent). And the problem is not limited to tonsillectomies. One of the most curious and unsettling facts about modern medicine is the variation in how often many procedures are done. Consider the figures for all surgical operations. By 1976 there were about half again as many done in Canada (per million people) as there were in England and Wales, and there were nearly half again as many in the United States as in Canada. These variations have persisted. Age and sex differences among the three countries might be thought a possible explanation – a country could have more old men in need of more prostate surgery, or more women who might need more hyster-ectomies – but the comparisons have been adjusted to take such differences into account, so that it is as if the countries had identical age and sex make-up.

Of course, different countries have different lifestyles, different diets, even to some extent different genes, so they could well have different rates of illness. More gall bladder problems, more gall bladder surgery. The three countries also have three different ways of paying for health care, so there are different incentives for surgeons to perform operations. These facts may help explain the international variations. But there is a more puzzling phenomenon. Differences *among* Can-adian provinces are as great or greater than the international differences;

so are the differences among states within the US. Nine of the ten Canadian provinces were studied from 1968 to 1977, and the variation was as large as for the three different countries.

As for variations within the US, a Rand Corporation study completed in 1986 counted surgical procedures in Medicare patients in thirteen geographical areas spread over eight states. The most consistent operation was hernia repair, which was only one and a half times more common in the place with the most operations than in the place with the fewest – or almost the proportion by which Canada exceeds England and Wales for all surgery. The operations with the largest place-to-place variation were total knee replacements (up to six-fold differences between the highest and lowest surgery rates), destruction of benign skin growths (up to eight-fold differences) and repair of an ailing hip (up to eleven-fold).

All of these comparisons are corrected for age and sex. A reasonable explanation for the widely differing rates of surgery would then seem to be regional differences in the rates of illnesses, and also the fact that, despite relatively uniform payment systems, some parts of Canada or the US are more advanced in standards of medical care than others. But there is more to the puzzle yet. Local variations *within* provinces and states are also very large. A study of forty-four counties in Ontario showed from two- to four-fold differences between the highest- and lowest-ranking counties for various kinds of surgery, with the exception of removal of part of the colon, which showed a surprising nine-fold difference.

Similar local variation exists in the UK and the US. Among twenty-one districts in the West Midlands alone, there was a one-and-a-half- to more than four-times difference in the rates at which each of seven kinds of operations were carried out – hernia repair, appendectomy, and removal of the gall bladder, prostate, uterus, tonsils or haemorrhoids. The region of New England shows a similar range of local variation for these seven operations, even though overall rates of surgery are much higher in New England than in old England. Hysterectomy, for instance, is about two and a half times more common in New England, yet the ratio of highest to lowest local rate – 2.1 to 1 in the West Midlands, 2.2 to 1 in New England – is almost identical. Even Norway, which was studied by the same investigators, and where the rates of most surgery are also far below those of New England, has similar within-country variation.

What are we to make of these strange numbers? Although some people have assumed that the high rates usually indicate better surgical practice – that the communities with lower rates are more backward medically and need to catch up – there is little evidence that this is generally true. On the contrary, there is growing evidence that for many types of surgery too many operations are done in some places; that is, in many instances the surgery was not only ineffective or harmful, but could have been predicted in advance to be so, on the basis of the patient's status and record.

Caesarian section is a case in point. Its frequency has risen over the last few decades in the UK, Canada and the US, but it is much the highest in the States, where – again, with lots of local variation – it accounts for around one fourth of all births. American physicians defending their practice cite the steady decline in infant mortality that accompanied the rise in Caesarian sections. However, since the UK and Canada have had similar declines in mortality with lower rates of Caesarian section, and have lower absolute mortality rates than the US, the association can be questioned. More compelling is the fact that Ireland, with an approach of carefully managed vaginal delivery, has experienced comparable declines in infant mortality in recent decades while keeping the Caesarian section rate down to around six per cent of births.

Germans, including doctors, seem to have a thing about the heart. Every culture has its folklore about health and illness, and for Germans the general tradition has been that if your heart is fine the rest of you will follow. Doctors thus tend to prescribe many different drugs for low blood pressure, a condition less likely to be thought of as an illness in other countries, and they very frequently prescribe digitalis, a medicine that strengthens the heartbeat, and that elsewhere is reserved for seriously weakened hearts. The Germans also have a tradition of sending patients to spas to convalesce in peaceful surroundings for a full six weeks after a heart attack, an approach that would strike American doctors, for example, as counterproductive – they would see it as putting a vigorous person who could be back in the stream of life out to pasture instead.

With this emphasis on caring for the heart, Doctor Jürgen Müller, an East Berlin radiologist specializing in heart and blood vessel imaging, viewed the 1989 collapse of the Berlin Wall with particular excitement. For most of his countrymen it meant an open gateway to freedom, the taste of potential prosperity and an unheard of new level of cultural richness. For Müller it meant all of that, plus a first-time ticket to the frontier of cardiology. The East had spent five per cent of its Gross Domestic Product on health care, the West nine – and with a larger per capita GDP. The East had no-frills medicine, the West had every conceivable new technological advance, fresh from the laboratory and factory. For the first time in his thirty years of practice, Doctor Müller began to look at his Western colleagues' equipment with something other than distant envy.

Ramin Radmanesh is hoping to give shape to Doctor Müller's longings. He is one of the sales representatives from Siemens, a West German firm that is a leading producer of medical technology in the world. Siemens would like to supply the state-of-the-art cardiac catheterization lab – with its equipment for making images of the insides of the arteries supplying the heart and for repairing some kinds of disease found there – that Müller would love to have to replace the broken-down old system he has used for seventeen years. But the Siemens people do not go in for hard-pressure sales. When Müller makes his first trip to the United States, where he attends the annual meeting of the Radiological Society of North America, Radmanesh guides the overwhelmed doctor around the equipment-filled exhibit hall, helping him find his way through the dazzling maze of competing products and brands.

According to medical company executives, the modern increase in life expectancy is due mainly to drugs and equipment. This is far from true; as shown by the late Thomas McKeown, a leading British authority on the history of health, among others, it is mainly due to economic, social and lifestyle changes, and to a lesser extent to specific preventive measures such as vaccines. Drugs and medical equipment compete for last place in importance. But in an almost twenty-first-century industrial society, it is understandable that some avid fans of technology would be hard put to see how change could come from anything else. Nevertheless, it does. And increasingly, hard-headed physicians and medical economists are proving that expensive advances on the frontier of technology – magnetic resonance imaging, for example, an elegant advance in making very detailed pictures of the inside of the body without the risks inherent in X-rays or CAT scanning, or the Siemens company's latest in cardiac catheterization – are over-used in a way that far exceeds their effectiveness, and relentlessly saps resources of a more modest kind that would make a much greater positive impact on health.

For Professor Lothar Heinemann, an East German epidemiologist who specializes in heart disease, the medical floodgates opened by the recent collapse of the Wall are not an unreserved blessing. 'I worry about the big-pocket medicine we are now implementing,' he says.

Before the Wall came down, we talked about preventing this development. Now it's here and we can't prevent it any more – we have to cope with the new procedures. Prevention needs to be more emphasized. But I am pretty sure both patients and doctors are mainly looking for big technology, what's new, fascinating, which is increasing the faith of the population in medicine. Doctors are great believers when new technology is being implemented. They believe there are only advantages for the patient, [but] the advantages are exaggerated.

Preventing the spread of lifesaving technology? Professor Heinemann speaks wistfully, even regretfully, about East Germany's technologically backward past. Is he some sort of anti-medicine Luddite trying to hold back the future, ready to smash the catheterization imagers turned out by Siemens? Hardly. In fact he is on the crest of a currently breaking worldwide wave that includes many of the most sophisticated thinkers in medicine. The men and women in white coats in the operating theatres and catheterization labs who scrub up and, without hesitation, do whatever supposedly needs to be done are considered the practical ones, but it is people like Heinemann – shifting their numbers around, making their calculations, scribbling their summaries – who turn out to be practical, while the 'doers' are often shown to be dreamers and bumblers. And these dreamy doers who may not really know what it is they are doing often have our lives in their hands.

Consider, for example, the over-enthusiasm for the artificial heart. The problem seemed simple: the heart is a pump; engineers make innumerable excellent working pumps, therefore we should be able to make a pump to replace the heart. In the United States, Utah was the focus of activity, and the Jarvik artificial heart was developed in Salt Lake City. There and elsewhere, heart transplants had been gaining credibility through increasingly evident effectiveness. But the dream of the manufactured heart remained: no donors, no thorny ethical questions, no supply snags, no tissue compatibility problems, just lovely heart machines gliding off the assembly line into the hands of the surgeon – and from there only a short way to the patient's waiting chest.

The only trouble was that the machines, once implanted, were not so lovely. They were vigorously rejected by the patients' immune systems as foreign tissue; and, lacking living tissue's ability to repair itself, they could not withstand the brutal burden of endless pumping that any live, healthy heart finds routine. They accumulated clots and built up cellular blockages as the body's immune system attacked this foreign object, while pounding themselves to breaking point trying to keep up the normal activities of life. Barney Clark, the middle-aged man who became the Jarvik's first patient, developed complications, was reoperated on, developed more complications, and finally succumbed. He was followed by one patient after another; they lived for a few months, or a year, or occasionally they survived for most of a second year.

Each case cost hundreds of thousands of pounds. Even physicians used to spending that kind of money and more were questioning whether the Jarvik heart was worth it. Finally in 1985 and again in 1988, special US government committees were convened to evaluate the procedure. Their conclusion was that public funds should no longer be used to support the programme. Despite strong advocacy by patients and their families, as well as by Congressional representatives from the state of Utah, government funding was withdrawn − tantamount to abandoning the programme − but this turned out to be temporary. Pressure from Congress, instigated by representatives of the state of Utah with no knowledge of the scientific and medical issues, led to resumption of the programme.

West German heart doctors continue to strive towards the goal of a completely implantable artificial heart. For Professor Heinemann, the sceptical East German epidemiologist, a success with it would be 'very important for a few persons at very high risk − it's a last hope for them. But for the majority, it is a loss of money and by the end I am sure a loss of health.'

Interestingly, the parallel process undergone by natural heart transplantation during the early 1980s produced what seemed at first glance to be the opposite outcome. Rejection of the new heart was largely subject to control, reoperation rates were satisfactorily low, and five-year survival rates climbed steadily to the point where the majority of patients − at least 65 per cent − were alive after five years. Today such statistics are still improving, and heart transplantation is a widely used and thoroughly accepted method of treatment, limited mainly by the number of hearts available.

But at second glance it still costs a fortune. Doctor Thomas Preston, a cardiologist at the University of Washington (Seattle) and historian of the field, has called the artificial heart programme an 'expensive, unsupervised experiment' that was properly suspended and should have been left at that. He warns that it is only the tip of an iceberg of similar problems, some just as costly, on which health care could founder. In fact, the modern history of surgery on the heart and blood vessels has shown one procedure after another to have been widely adopted before they were proved effective, and that procedures were used in the end on many patients for whom they were not appropriate. Some of these operations, in fact, should not have been carried out on anyone at all.

Take, for instance, surgery on the carotid artery and its branches, which are among the most important vessels supplying blood to the brain. (The carotid is the artery that gives you a pulse next to your windpipe.) A lifetime of bad habits, especially excessive intake of saturated fats, will cause fatty growths to develop in the artery, especially at its branching point high in the throat. These blockages reduce blood flow to the brain, and may cause dizziness, blackouts, or perhaps only a noise heard by a doctor holding a stethoscope to the throat – a little whooshing sound made by blood squeezing through a narrow space. As with the artificial heart, the simple facts of the plumbing made the solution seem obvious: go around the clogged stretch of artery.

A logical way of doing this was devised, using a less important artery from outside the brain – the one that gives you the pulse in your temple – and inserting it where it could supply the brain, or 'cranium', directly.

The procedure was named the extracranial-intracranial or EC-IC bypass operation. It seemed so logical that reports of its success with individual patients caused more and more surgeons to do the procedure on more and more patients, until it was being done thousands of times a year in the US alone. The only drawback seemed to be that there was no real proof that it worked. So neurologist Doctor Henry Barnett of London, Ontario, led a large international study that randomly assigned nearly 1400 patients – around a third of them in Europe, including some in Manchester, England, and around a fifth in Asia, mainly Japan – to be treated either with drugs or with the EC-IC bypass operation. The result was very hard for many doctors to believe: there was no advantage to surgery.

Barnett and his colleagues' study had to weather a storm of controversy lasting for years, but in the end the EC-IC bypass suffered a fate similar to that met, at least temporarily, by the artificial heart: the US government ceased to pay for it. As Doctor Barnett put it, 'This stunning reversal of what everybody thought made a lot of people think that a lot of surgical procedures had to be evaluated with controlled studies. I think it was in that way, for those of us involved with the nervous system, a bit of a landmark study. It taught us that we simply couldn't go on believing that what we were doing was right without proving it.'

But the question remains: how could hundreds of surgeons

throughout the world have been permitted to do an operation thousands of times a year if it had not been properly tested first? The answer is distressingly simple. There is no procedure for formally scrutinizing operations or diagnostic tests, unless they involve new substances. In Britain the Committee on Safety of Medicines and in the US the Food and Drug Administration have a mandate to, among other things, run studies of new drugs to determine that they are one, safe, and two, more effective for the stated purpose than placebo. Such legal standards do not exist for new operations or new diagnostic tests, except to the extent that they involve new substances; their adoption or rejection is left to the judgement of experienced practitioners.

The threat of being sued for malpractice has made practitioners, particularly in the US, even less willing to be out on a limb alone, doing an operation or test few others have adopted. There is an old saying in medicine that you should not be the first or the last to use a new drug or procedure. But being part of the medical crowd is no assurance against doing harm if the crowd's collective judgement is based more on enthusiasm than evidence. In fact, after a certain critical mass of doctors in your area have adopted the practice in question, you can be more legally vulnerable by shunning it – this is true of Caesarian sections, for example – since the 'standard of practice' you will be measured against in a court of law is precisely what those colleagues are currently doing. Even where threat of legal action is not as powerful, as in Britain, doctors feel the natural group pressure to conform, to go along with fashions which seem particularly appealing at the time and for which rational justifications can be made. The result is that there can be a sea-change in practice, a widespread adoption of a new procedure, without clear evidence that it works.

The infamous frontal lobotomy is perhaps the worst example of this kind, though not the only one. Egas Moniz, a Portuguese neurologist known for discovering the technique for imaging brain blood vessels, developed in 1936 a way of severing the connections between the frontal lobes and the brain's emotional centres. It was a startlingly simple procedure that seemed to have an almost magical calming effect on psychotic and other mentally disturbed patients. Moniz emphasized that it should not be used except where all other methods had failed, but its use spread rapidly despite this warning. In one version it could be done as an almost routine procedure in the doctor's surgery: a slender blade was introduced through the bony case of the eye deep within the skull and rotated back and forth to slice through the brain's wiring. The procedure's popularity grew steadily, and many thousands of such operations were done. Thirteen years after its invention, in

1949, its prestige was such that Moniz shared the Nobel Prize in medicine for inventing it.

But it was about to be almost completely discredited. During the 1950s many studies of patients who had been subjected to the procedure revealed that their mental and emotional lives had been severely impaired, to the extent that whatever the calming effects, they could not justify the irrepairable damage done in most cases. Indeed, the word lobotomized became synonymous with a devastating loss of ability and identity. The number of lobotomies performed went from thousands a year to none in less than a decade. And the doctors who had done them quietly retired or turned their talents to other methods.

Lobotomies came and went even more dramatically but in essentially the same way as the tonsillectomy fad during those decades, and the hysterectomy fad a little later: credulous doctors sent their patients to over-confident surgeons, whose standards of practice were shaped by colleagues' anecdotes and by their own experience rather than by rigorous scientific research. To institute controls to help prevent such surgical fads has, however, proved difficult.

In the States, the Office of Technology Assessment of the US Congress and the Institute of Medicine of the US National Academy of Sciences have been attempting for years to design mechanisms for the systematic evaluation of medical technology, just as drugs are evaluated by the Food and Drug Administration. But these efforts have been regularly hampered by recent Presidents on the advice of some physicians and other members of the health care 'industry'. Yet in Britain, where the profit motive in health care is not such an issue, there has also been a slow response to the need for an evaluation system. The medical literature has carried many proposals for reform, and one can envisage a British Committee on Safety of Surgery resembling the long-established Committee on Safety of Medicines. Such a committee would presumably establish a procedure's effectiveness in animals, and follow with randomized, controlled human trials – under ethical supervision comparable to that in drug trials.

The difficulty in establishing official controls underscores how intrinsic to modern medicine is the technological imperative and the concept of the easy surgical fix. It also points up people's reluctance to participate in randomized trials; rather than frankly recognizing that the choice is a toss up, and participate in an experiment for the advancement of medical knowledge, we encourage our doctors to exaggerate their degree of confidence in a given procedure, so we can choose it wholeheartedly for ourselves.

And what fads might we be in the midst of today? Caesarian

section? Prostate gland removal? Surgery for low back pain? We just don't know. For these procedures and a dismaying number of others there have been no rigorously controlled scientific studies to serve as the foundation for the practice. Doctors believe in these procedures because people have a good chance of coming through them successfully. But there are no studies to answer the obvious question: how much worse off would they have been without the operation? And the next: is that enough to justify the risk, the discomfort and the cost of the surgery?

Although most cardiac operations have fared better than artificial heart surgery, and although some have been almost miraculous – the correction of otherwise fatal congenital defects, for example, which has given countless children their lives through deft, quick snipping and sewing – the field has certainly had its share of fiascos. The Beck operation, for instance, was designed to relieve angina – heart pain usually caused by reduced blood supply in an artery blocked by fatty growths called plaques. Doctor Claude Beck, a surgeon, reasoned that if the thirsty heart muscle was deliberately injured, new blood vessels would grow into it and resupply it with blood. The procedure was to strip off the top layer of heart muscle and then scrape it with asbestos, irritating it until it was bloody. In a 1958 article in the *Journal of the American Medical Association*, Beck claimed a ninety-seven per cent success rate in relieving heart pain.

Actually, there was no more real scientific evidence for the procedure's success then than there is now, when the operation has been long abandoned for lack of such evidence. But the way it developed remains instructive. Patients with angina often suffer extreme, crushing pain, which usually emerges with the physical exertion needed to live a normal life – climbing a flight of stairs, say, or walking to the shops. The pain, too, is often the harbinger of a heart attack, that final destruction of cardiac muscle that has been starved for blood for too long, destruction that all too often results in death. Faced by the plight of such patients, it is understandable that doctors in the early to mid-twentieth century – a time when the number of heart attacks rose enormously – were almost desperately searching for something, anything, that might relieve the problem. And as an old medical saying goes, desperate maladies require desperate remedies.

The Beck operation was not the most desperate. In France in 1922 a surgeon tried the expedient of cutting the nerve that carried anginal pain from the heart to the brain. This seems a bizarre tactic, since it would destroy the early warning system which, by telling the brain to slow the body down, could often prevent a heart attack. But the severity of the pain has to be appreciated, and how hopeless advanced cases were in 1922. Today a surgeon may cut nerves in a dying cancer patient to relieve pain, knowing that the treatment is destructive but using it as a last resort to mitigate horrible suffering. That was the spirit in which angina was treated by severing a vital nerve. Another procedure involved removal of the thyroid gland in an effort to reduce heart stimulation by hormones, an operation which, by causing all the symptoms of thyroid deficiency, did more harm than good.

These procedures for angina always made some kind of physiological sense. One might say that they suffered from too much convincing scientific theory and not enough practical scientific proof. Another operation that became popular in the late 1940s was called internal mammary ligation. This meant tying off some important arteries in the chest wall in the hope of shunting extra blood towards the heart. By the late 1950s articles in medical journals reported relief of angina by this procedure in one-third to two-thirds of the cases.

However, the surgeons reporting these results had ignored an elementary rule of science: compare your experimental group with a control group. A team of cardiologists at the University of Washington in Seattle led by Doctor Leonard Cobb decided to do just that. Seventeen patients agreed to undergo surgery considered experimental; eight of them underwent internal mammary ligation, but the other nine went through the whole procedure except the tying off of the arteries. The results were published in the *New England Journal of Medicine* in 1959. Remarkably, the nine sham-operated controls (no longer allowable under today's ethical standards) received as much benefit from the surgery as the ones who had actually had their arteries tied off. They experienced reduction of pain, took fewer nitroglycerine tablets to control their angina, resumed normal activity and even had improvements in their electrocardiogram tracings – all to the same extent as those who got the full operation.

The Cobb study was a very small one, but it certainly called attention to the basic flaw in studies that merely reported the results for patients operated on, without a comparison control group. A powerful placebo effect could result from real or fake operations, presumably due to an enormous reduction of anxiety after undergoing surgery believed to be helpful. This effect, along with the natural ups and downs of a disease like angina even without any treatment at all, should have left physicians and surgeons sceptical of glowing reports – of the ninety-seven per cent success rate with the Beck asbestos procedure, for example.

But little such scepticism emerged. Arthur Vineberg, a Canadian surgeon reporting in leading medical journals in the late 1950s and 1960s, claimed success for a procedure even more drastic than Beck's. He took one of the same internal mammary arteries that would have been tied off in the earlier ligation procedure, and tried to divert it so that it would supply the heart muscle instead. An incision was made in the heart and a cut mammary artery was turned and sewed into the wound. The hope was that it would actually generate some normal branching and a new blood supply.

Subsequent studies of dogs and pigs showed that this rarely happened, but the Vineberg operation continued to be used throughout the 1960s, based on journal articles about uncontrolled trials – in effect, series of patients who were reported improved after the operation, but who were not compared to randomly assigned controls. By the early 1970s a group of medical scientists was poised to do a proper controlled trial of the Vineberg and Beck procedures. But by then both operations were being replaced by a new procedure – once again, based on weak evidence – that was sweeping cardiology: coronary artery bypass surgery. This operation was supremely logical, involving the replacement of clogged arteries with segments taken from unclogged arteries and veins elsewhere in the body. It awaited two important developments of the 1960s: the heart-lung machine, to do the work of the heart while it was under the knife; and truly effective imaging of the coronary arteries.

By 1975 about 60 000 bypass operations were done each year in the United States; by 1987 about 230 000. Most of these years went by before the results of randomized controlled trials of 'cabbage' – the surgeons' slang pronunciation of CABG, for Coronary Artery Bypass Graft – were available. Two large American trials, the Veterans Administration Cooperative Study and the Coronary Artery Surgery Study, whose results appeared during the mid-1980s, showed no difference in survival between angina patients who were randomly assigned to have the operation and those whom chance assigned to drug and other non-surgical treatments only. A large multi-centre trial in Europe, the European Coronary Surgery Study, found about a ten per cent greater five-year survival in the CABG group than in the group that had no surgery. But even this was disappointing for such a highly touted operation.

Heart surgeons responded by saying that the quality of the surgery in the trials was not high enough, that the patients were not sick enough and that pain reduction, for which surgery was successful in the trials, is a legitimate goal distinct from that of lengthening life. Their first point, if true, was partly moot; the average patient is not likely to be operated on by the very best surgeons in the world so we need to know how well things work when done by less exalted hands.

Their second point was accurate, and has led to practical consequences: today only the sickest patients – those with blockage of the largest coronary artery, the left main, or of three other arteries to the heart – go directly to bypass surgery, since these patients clearly benefit in terms of survival. Their third point was also valid: randomized controlled trials have proved the benefit of surgery over drug treatment in most categories of patients when the key measure is not mortality but pain. Critics of bypass surgery tend to discount the impact on pain in the absence of an impact on survival, an omission that is unfair to many suffering patients.

But while these guidelines for when bypass grafting should really be done were still being worked out, the operation was done tens of thousands of times unnecessarily – at least by today's standards. If CABG had been a new medication, the Committee on Safety of Medicines in Britain, or equivalent official national bodies, would have put it through systematic testing, including large randomized controlled trials, before it could be brought into such widespread use. (Even this, as we have seen, does not necessarily prevent widespread abuse.) But since it was a surgical operation, CABG could be widely carried out before such testing, and proper controlled trials had to catch up with practice. The same is true for all procedures as *procedures*. The recent debate over breast-augmentation surgery, for example, hinged on the damage done by silicone, a foreign chemical brought into the body, and not on the surgery itself. Substances are regulated, operations are not, and although this may be on the verge of change, it has not changed yet.

During the 1980s another procedure, PTCA, or 'pizza' – percutaneous transluminal coronary angioplasty – joined the ranks of heart treatments that spread widely before they were properly tested. PTCA has revolutionized the treatment of angina because it is in effect an operation that is not an operation. It is an extension of the technique for imaging arteries in the heart: a long thin tube is introduced through the body's blood vessels into the coronary arteries, but instead of a dye being released to show up on an X-ray film, a tiny balloon is inflated within the clogged artery, and the compromised channel is widened. The patient may be awake, and may even be sent home shortly after the angioplasty. Best of all from the viewpoint of the cardiologist, angioplasty can be learned and done by that same doctor, with no need for referral to a surgeon.

As the trials of CABG began to show that patients with only one-

or two-vessel obstruction were not living longer after their bypass operations, it became routine to send many of these less sick patients to PTCA (one of the rare situations in which pizza seems healthier than cabbage!). Yet the scientific evidence even for this decision is not sufficient to show that it is routinely the right one. Recent research suggests that there is an excess use of angioplasties that may rival the excess use of bypass grafts. It is clear that some patients' arteries close up again within months or years of the procedure, and the long-term effects remain uncertain. Accordingly, research trials are under way in the US, Britain, Germany and other European countries. But the frequency with which angioplasty is done shows no signs of slowing its rise to wait for the results.

Still another technique, rotoblation, has been catching on in both Britain and the United States. A tiny, diamond-studded brass burr attached to a flexible wire is introduced into the blocked artery in much the same way as an angioplasty balloon, but unlike the latter, it can be used in curved sections of arteries and other tight spots. The burr is rotated on the wire at high speed, like a dentist's drill. Early evidence suggests that it causes no damage to flexible tissues like the normal blood vessel wall, yet when it engages the hardened, calcium-filled plaque of atherosclerosis, it wears it down impressively, widening the channel. Unlike the balloon, it can even be used to reopen a channel in an artery completely blocked by calcified, fatty plaque. As one of several new technologies meant to improve on the balloon technique, it points up the difficulties for any evaluation system in keeping up with a dynamic research frontier.

Cardiologists on both sides of the Atlantic showed great enthusiasm for the rotoblator, and maybe it will prove to be the miracle cure for coronary artery disease that its promoters believe it to be. But once again, randomized trials lagged behind practice; no trials have as yet compared rotoblation to angioplasty, coronary bypass or, certainly, medical management – treatment with drugs, diet, exercise and other non-surgical approaches. Due to technical defects, the rotoblator was recently withdrawn from the market. And medical management is also changing. Several new drugs introduced for the lowering of cholesterol have recently been shown actually to widen arteries clogged by fatty plaques.

Moreover, changes in diet and lifestyle alone – without drugs or surgery – have also been shown capable of reducing the clogging of arteries. Most interesting of all, these effects will be permanent if the lifestyle changes are carried on, while the relief provided by the more dramatic procedures – bypass or angioplasty, cabbage or pizza – is temporary in most cases, lasting at most five to ten years. Ironically perhaps, none of the currently popular procedures has been proved superior to cholesterol-lowering drugs or mere lifestyle changes in increasing the blood supply to a thirsty heart.

In a place called Jackson Hole, Wyoming, where the pines seem to touch the sky and the Rocky Mountains range north and south for many hundreds of miles – 'Skyline Route' is the mailing address – Doctor David Eddy practises his medical specialty. He no longer wields a stethoscope or scalpel; his main tools now are a computer, some equations, exceptionally clear thought and carefully chosen words. And his one and only patient is medicine, especially in America but, by association, in much of the rest of the modern world.

The condition is far from hopeless, but it is alarming. It seems that the patient has indulged in lifelong habits that stand in the way of optimum health. The symptoms are bloated costs, acute malpractice litigation, weakening satisfaction and faltering respect. And the habits? Always insisting on doing something rather than nothing; unwillingness to recognize and concede uncertainty; over-reliance on received medical wisdom; and, worst of all, a persistent failure to study properly the outcomes of the things doctors routinely do. Doctor Eddy remains optimistic, pointing out that the patient has lived through many crises, often emerging stronger. But he is worried about the patient's overconfidence, which he rightly sees as a major obstacle to any future change.

Doctor Eddy embarked on his present career after dropping out of a prestigious training programme in cardiovascular surgery. A man with an intellectual as well as a mathematical bent, he began reviewing the evidence in favour of the procedures he was learning in his apprenticeship. He wanted to understand the science on which these operations were based, and he discovered that in many cases there wasn't any – at least none that was convincing. Randomized controlled trials, the gold standard of medical experimentation, had simply never been done to test the value of most procedures in his chosen field, procedures he was being taught and would be doing for the rest of his career. Dismayed by this lack of evidence, he decided to study the mathematical tools for making decisions and for assessing the outcomes of those decisions; he dropped out of the surgical residency, and eventually he acquired a PhD in outcomes analysis to go along with his MD. Since then he has carried forward the work of John Wennberg and others, asking tough, relentless questions about why doctors do what they do.

In a series of hard-hitting columns in the *Journal of the American Medical Association* over the past few years, Eddy has expressed sympathy for the situation of practising physicians – but not so much that he fails to let them know that they are wasting billions of dollars and subjecting millions of patients to unproven, possibly harmful procedures. One of the laws I was taught in medical school was: when you don't know what to do, don't do anything. This, it seems, is the hardest rule of all for the modern physician. It was easier for nineteenth-century physicians, since there was not very much they could do anyway; so they watched and waited and comforted and, when they could, relieved pain as the illness took its course.

But in the mid-twentieth century physicians began understandably to feel a certain confidence in being able to change the course of illness, and often to turn illness into health. Antibiotics counter some diseases, surgery many others. Techniques of imaging made it possible to see right through the body, not in vague shadows but in precise detail. Increasingly complex chemistry laboratories offered scores, then hundreds of different measurements. Blood could be safely replaced, then the heart and the kidney could be bypassed by dazzling machines, and finally those same organs could be lifted out when disease struck and replaced with new and better ones. Every day, in every medical practice, people who would previously have been crippled or dead were sent home to go on with their normal lives. Is it any wonder that doctors became a little too sure of themselves?

Medical advances have continued, but not all of them are equally effective, and the 'miraculous' cures – 'jewels strewn on the landscape waiting for us to pick them up,' was how one old heart surgeon described them to me in 1980 – became fewer and farther between. Each generation of antibiotics came to the limits of its usefulness as microbes evolved and adapted, and new drugs were needed just to maintain past gains. Obviously needed operations like the removal of deadly cancers and the rebuilding of malformed infant hearts were boldly instituted, and worked; but many other operations came and went, and some that remained in common practice had a value, if any, that was not so easy to prove. New technologies of measurement and imaging were everywhere in great demand; they often provided advantages over older, cheaper methods, but few physicians or patients asked whether the added value was great enough to justify the cost.

Doctor Eddy puts it more strongly:

In fact very little of medicine has been carefully evaluated in well designed, well controlled studies. It's really quite amazing, but after hundreds of years, I would estimate that only about ten to twenty per cent of medical practices have been evaluated properly. What that means for the patient – and not just the patient but for the physician – is that for a large proportion of practices we really don't know what the outcomes or what the effects are.

The momentum generated by truly great medical advances served to keep the system moving and confident even at times when the advances were small, or perhaps non-existent. Thus each new and costly medication had to prove itself only against placebos, not against tried and true, less expensive drugs. Procedures like coronary bypass and angioplasty worked and were needed sometimes, but in many advanced countries (not including Britain, as yet) each operation was done thousands of times more often a year than was necessary at an unacceptable level of cost and risk. Magnetic resonance scans slipped into common use; they were better for some purposes than the widely used CAT scan, but they were not three times better, although they cost three times more.

Under the 'what-if-it's-your-mother' principle, these declining ratios of benefit to cost are not an issue; if the treatment helps at all, or even if it *might* help, you want it. You don't want the doctor to stand there and do nothing. In fact, you and the doctor may share in a barely conscious collusion: 'no evidence that it works' is subtly transformed into 'well, it might work' and then into 'sure, it's worth a try.' *We can't just do nothing* haunts both patient and doctor when faced by not knowing what to do.

According to David Eddy, very often you can, and should, and must do nothing, painful as it may be. Every time you do something medically unjustified, you expose a patient to needless risk; and in a world of limited resources, you may also be denying another patient a treatment that really will work, because the resource has been used for something needless.

Eddy is devoting his life to raising the consciousness of doctors about these simple facts. But his programme faces formidable obstacles. Ignorance and greed are merely the obvious ones. Much the hardest are the need felt to *do* something; the what-if-it's-your-mother rule; the persistence of medical custom, sometimes idiosyncratic or even irrational; the lingering impact of outdated training; the medical equivalents of fads and fashions; pressure from patients to have the latest and the best; and the misplaced confidence of some doctors, dazzled by the history of their science, and insufficiently sceptical of the power in their hands. These factors are not confined to the States;

most of them operate, if to a lesser extent, in Britain and elsewhere.

The remedy Eddy offers is called practice policies. These are guidelines for physicians as to what they should do in various given clinical situations. They may be set by local or national physicians' organizations, by corporate employers of physicians, by hospital boards, by insurance companies or by governments. What they have in common is their basis on outcome studies, ideally on randomized controlled trials, but at worst on careful statistics documenting what has actually been done for and to patients and, above all, what the outcomes were.

Outcomes can be defined in many different ways. Death is an outcome, but so is pain; the rate of blood flow through an artery, the strength of a stream of urine, the force of a breath, the dosage of nitroglycerine pills needed, the number of return visits to the doctor, the continued enjoyment of sex – all these are outcomes. For a distressingly large number of common medical and surgical procedures – most, according to some serious studies – we do not know what the outcomes are. We cannot therefore design rational practice policies. Many obstacles stand in the way of such studies, but the first step on this journey is to recognize that the studies have yet to be done.

The willingness of ordinary people – patients, you and me – to participate in such studies, including random assignment to different treatments of uncertain value, is fundamental. As Doctor Tudor Hart has put it, 'If we want to benefit from real medical knowledge, we should also contribute to it.' If we face up to the uncertainties that really exist in medicine, we can appreciate that allowing ourselves to be part of a randomized trial is no great sacrifice, because – and this is the whole point – *no one knows* which of the experimental groups we may land in by chance is really better, if either is. Indeed, there are now sophisticated mathematical techniques for determining as early as possible in the study if and when one of the choices has in fact proved better. At that point the study can be cut short – this has been done in several recent experiments, including a study of low-dose aspirin in reducing heart attacks – and *all* participants in the study can take advantage of the new treatment, whose value they themselves have helped to prove.

What we do sacrifice is a sense of control, a full-force belief in the effectiveness of what is being done to avert the threat posed by the illness. That could mean a sacrifice of the placebo effect – which, as we know, can be an important part of the treatment. Not everyone can be called on to make this sacrifice, especially not everyone facing a life-threatening illness. This is what is missing from Doctor Eddy's otherwise excellent formulation. One could say that is *too* rational; in fact a completely rational analysis must take into account the irrational element in human affairs and in medicine. Perhaps it was because he was disturbed by this paradox that Doctor Eddy dropped out of clinical medicine. As every practising clinician knows, the irrational is an inescapable part of every doctor-patient encounter – and as we have seen in Chapter 1, not by any means an undesirable one. Without an intense desire to help – one that occasionally must go too far – we would have no doctors at all.

Nevertheless, every doctor, if not every patient, should be capable of a planned pause in the battle against illness, during which a fully rational analysis can be focused on what he or she is doing. As Doctor Tudor Hart has written, 'Good doctors are those who are prepared to measure, or let others measure, how bad they are; or, more constructively, are prepared to accept that their work can be convincingly improved only if they are prepared to start by measuring its outcomes, errors and omissions.'

Doctor Caldwell Esselstyn Jr of the Cleveland Clinic is an extraordinary man. Among other accomplishments, he won an Olympic Gold Medal for rowing in 1956, and served in a field hospital in Vietnam in 1966-67, not to mention making numerous contributions in the approach to breast cancer and thyroid surgery. But like Doctor Eddy, he has begun to question some long-accepted surgical wisdom. Although he continues to operate for many purposes, he too has found another activity that he considers more important, as he argued in 'Beyond Surgery', his 1991 presidential address to the American Association of Endocrine Surgeons.

His new mission has not taken him away from patients; on the contrary, he is often surrounded by them, even in his home. There, together, they partake in meals that have the power not only to prevent, but to reverse the atherosclerosis of the arteries that causes anginal pain, heart attack and many strokes. We now know that all the operations invented over the years to treat this condition, including some recent ones that seem to work rather well, can usually be avoided if the patient goes on an anti-atherosclerotic diet.

That means a diet low in saturated fat and cholesterol, with adequate fibre and complex carbohydrate. Before Doctor Esselstyn presumed to put his patients on the diet, he put himself on it, to find out if he could lower his blood cholesterol to below 150 (UK: 3.90). This level is considered by most physicians to be almost unreachable, although throughout the world rural people living on traditional diets have often had cholesterol levels in that neighbourhood. So in fact it is far from impossible; it really means returning to a pattern once common everywhere, and only considered so difficult because we have become accustomed to dangerously rich, fatty foods.

Doctor Esselstyn succeeded in lowering his own cholesterol level to less than 150. Having found that he could do it without ceasing to enjoy food, he proceeded to apply the same principles to patients – the sickest patients the cardiologists could send him. These patients, as a result of his simple good care and diet, have avoided surgery that they had been assured was essential. Some have had serious problems. But that makes them as a group no worse off, and probably better off, than they would have been if sent to surgery. Although there was no control group in Doctor Esselstyn's research, others are doing carefully controlled studies.

For example, Doctor Dean Ornish, along with colleagues at the University of California at San Francisco and the University of Texas Medical School in Houston, is conducting a study known as the Lifestyle Heart Trial. Forty-one patients with serious coronary artery disease were randomly assigned to one of two groups. Twenty-two patients in the experimental group followed an extremely low-fat diet, walked half an hour a day and attended two four-hour stress-reduction sessions a week. Nineteen in the control group followed their regular doctors' orders – which included some reduction of fat intake and some exercise. Patients were given angiograms – X-rays of their coronary arteries – and PET scans to document the clogging of their arteries, which was substantial before the study started, markedly increasing their risk of heart attack.

The study will follow patients for four years and is still in progress, but according to a report in the distinguished British journal, *The Lancet*, the experimental group was doing much better than the control group after one year. Eighteen of the twenty-two patients showed significant reduction of the blockage in their arteries. Three more showed slight reduction and only one, who failed to comply with the experimental regimen, showed a worsening of blockage. As a group they claimed a ninety-one per cent reduction in the frequency of chest pains. But the control group reported a major increase in chest pains, and on the more objective measure of blockage in the arteries, ten of the nineteen had worsened.

Doctor Claude L'Enfant, director of the US government's National Heart, Lung and Blood Institute, a mainstream institution, said that the Ornish study 'offers strong scientific evidence that lifestyle changes alone can actually reverse' clogging of the coronary arteries, 'without the use of cholesterol-lowering drugs'. Doctor Alexander Leaf, professor of medicine at Harvard Medical School, has said emphatically of Ornish's approach, 'We can't go on merely buying a little time by doing bypasses and angioplasty, but having the disease continue to worsen, when you can reverse the disease with these methods.'

The Lifestyle study has been criticized because of its small sample, and it has been pointed out that many patients would probably find it very hard to comply with the diet involved. But both Doctor Ornish's patients and Doctor Esselstyn's have actually complied quite well, probably because considerable effort in each case went into creating a diet that was palatable as well as healthy.

Although most physicians would sneer at these doctors' involvement with something as simple as diet, they have in a real sense cured a small number of people of coronary artery disease, something that has never been done with bypass surgery, angioplasty, rotoblation, or any other surgical technique known to science – all these being more or less clumsy repair jobs that figuratively as well as literally bypass the underlying disease process. Dr Esselstyn has made most of his patients essentially heart-attack proof, if not permanently at least long enough so that they may live to die of something else.

As he points out, none of the impressive mechanical techniques addresses the fundamental molecular, biochemical disorder involved in heart disease, while diet certainly does. Yet despite the great emphasis on molecular science in medical school, little is taught about diet, one of the most powerful ways of changing the molecular processes of the body. Heart diseases are the leading killers in industrialized nations, exceeding all cancers and thoroughly dwarfing a so far comparatively minor problem such as AIDS. Yet they are almost completely preventable, and most are effectively treatable, with dietary measures. In the last few years carefully designed studies have proved the effectiveness of diet and other lifestyle changes in shrinking the growths blocking arteries supplying the heart.

So why are there so few Esselstyns when there are thousands of bypass surgeons and angioplasters? Because neither medical science, nor medical education, nor health care economics have caught up with the facts of life and death as they are affected by diseases of the arteries. Because the technological imperative and the profit motive have dazzled physicians, hospital corporations and health insurers. And also, certainly, because patients – people in general – have relentlessly insisted on abdicating responsibility for their own health and their own treatment, choosing in almost every case the quick fix, only to be bitterly disappointed when the quick fix doesn't really work.

CHAPTER 6

DISORDERED
STATES

Psychiatry has long been medicine's neglected stepchild. Throughout most of European history the mentally ill – certainly those with serious disorders – were looked upon as demonic or, at the least, 'possessed' by demons. An unsympathetic, superstitious populace confronted them with a mixture of fear and contempt. At worst, they were ritually 'tried' and done away with as witches or heretics; at best, they were permanently locked away, in places where their care was poor enough to ensure that they would not live very long. Beset by psychic pain – pain that those close to it deem terrible and terrifying, perhaps worse than almost any form of physical suffering – they had their raw emotional wounds relentlessly made worse by the responses of the ignorant world around them, and they were subject to physical illnesses that gave embodiment to their suffering.

In the late nineteenth century scientific views of mental illness began to prevail over primitive religious ones, but there was still little scientists or physicians could do. Indeed science proved as inhumane as any religious zealotry. The early twentieth century saw a rise of eugenic ideas about the mentally ill which led to laws that authorized the sterilization of the mentally ill in the United States and their actual extermination in 1930s Germany. In the late 1930s and 1940s science produced the frontal lobotomy, which 'calmed' the mentally ill at the cost of serious damage to mind and personality. By mid-century, when the dismal failure of lobotomies was apparent, we were back to the strait-jacket and padded cell – anything to prevent a psychotic from harming someone, most likely himself. Such methods are hard to think of as humane, unless one is faced by a seriously mentally disturbed person intent on self-damage. By this time too, psychoanalysis had spread throughout the Western world, but it had little to offer the most seriously ill, who dwelt in a delusional world of psychotic thought, unreachable with psychotherapy.

In the 1950s the situation changed dramatically. Jean Delay and Pierre Deniker, two psychiatrists in France, discovered that chlorpromazine, a drug used against nausea, had the effect of blocking the thought disorders of schizophrenics, even in the absence of general sedation. The consequences were stunning. Within a few years of the discovery, psychotic patients throughout the world who had known only incarceration and restraint began to function well enough and safely enough to be discharged. Certainly, they still needed supervision and care, especially to try to ensure that they continued to take their medicine. But many of them could be set free at last from the institutional settings to which their illnesses had confined them and others like them since the dawn of civilization.

As it became clear that at least a partly independent life would now be possible for many schizophrenics, some observers began to believe that it should be mandatory. Mental institutions were widely seen more as centres of confinement, even punishment, than of treatment, and in some quarters it was taken for granted that institutionalization was always and everywhere bad for patients, something that psychiatrists and hospital administrators did for their own benefit. Independent life for these patients began to be seen as a civil liberties issue, not primarily a medical one.

This in fact was a tribute to the success of chlorpromazine and other related anti-psychotic drugs. By 1975 almost two-thirds of the resident patients in American mental hospitals – more than 300 000 people – had been discharged, and a similar development followed in Britain and elsewhere. For a time this was seen as something unreservedly positive, but it turned out that the history of neglect of the mentally ill was not over. They were no longer mainly incarcerated and ignored; now they were mainly discharged and ignored. Anti-psychotic drugs were a boon, but no cure. The thousands who were discharged needed many kinds of support – nursing homes, halfway houses, job training programmes, day care, family therapy, and frequent contacts with well-trained nurses, social workers, psychologists and psychiatrists. They needed to be medically monitored for the neurological disorders that ten to twenty per cent of them develop as a side-effect of the drugs they take, or in the case of lithium, for blood levels of the drug and for rare but catastrophic blood disorders. Although

diagnosis and medication were improving steadily, most of these com-
monsense support services were not available, and did not become
available as time went by. Some of those that did appear were so
inferior that conditions for patients were worse there than in residential
institutions – and sometimes much worse, not excluding physical
cruelty and dangerous neglect.

But the American taxpayers who had been willing to pay a small
fortune to keep a schizophrenic incarcerated were apparently not
willing to spend considerably less to maintain the same person in a
decent and safe situation outside the hospital. The result was that many
thousands of mentally ill people became homeless wanderers, tramps
and bag ladies, vulnerable to involvement with alcohol and illicit drugs
that could only worsen their illnesses, and generally living in a marginal
way in which they are neither properly stabilized on anti-psychotic
drugs nor quite bad enough to be reinstitutionalized – at least not
more than occasionally. Pathetically vulnerable to crime and abuse,
persistently dangerous to themselves if not to others, they are in a
situation where the mental hospital may often be a boon, and may
indeed be the closest thing they will ever have to a home. It is estimated
that at least a quarter of all the homeless in America have a serious
mental illness, and around half of those appear to have schizophrenia.
Looking at it from the other side, one recent study in Kansas found
that forty per cent of hospitalized mental patients had no home to go
to if and when they were discharged.

In Britain the concept of community care has been widely touted
as the answer to caring for the mentally ill, and other groups, previously
based in hospitals or institutions. But initial enthusiasm has given way
to increasing doubts, and problems similar to the States, including lack
of both financial and professional resources, are beginning to emerge.
As in the States, but to a lesser extent, the policy of closing down
psychiatric hospitals is coming under question because the support
system for the patients discharged is often proving inadequate.

Doctor Jack Gorman, director of a clinical research ward for
psychiatric patients at New York's distinguished Columbia Pres-
byterian Hospital, regards deinstitutionalization as a failure.

> I take in very few homeless schizophrenics because I have nowhere
> for them to go at the end of their three-month stay. The mandate for
> my programme is that they must have somewhere to go that can
> sustain them, before I can take them on. It must be remembered that
> there is no cure for schizophrenia . . . All [the drugs] have side-effects.
> The big problem remains the lack of a support system.

For those lucky enough to fulfil Doctor Gorman's mandate, he provides the most modern, comprehensive care. That includes a carefully selected spectrum of the latest anti-psychotic drugs, subtly monitored for side-effects in individual patients; an accepting, supportive milieu on the ward, where patients get help and understanding from others with parallel illnesses, as well as structured activities and professional intervention; and perhaps above all, discharge to a stable environment, either in a halfway house that continues needed professional care, or in a family able to make the sacrifices and provide the kind of support that can at least postpone a further breakdown. And, importantly, an environment that encourages the person in question to continue taking the medicine.

Maggie, a patient of Doctor Gorman's, resembles most psychotics the world over in believing that what she experiences is totally real, and she accordingly resents the people taking care of her for denying her reality. 'I'm stuck here with voices that they will not tell me what to do about because they believe them to not be real. I believe them to be real people and it doesn't go away for me.' She feels she would be better off with people who could see things her way.

'I really don't know if I can be helped merely with medication. I think my life situation is a struggle and a dangerous one, and I'm fighting for my life sometimes ... If I even ask for help, people say, "I don't know where you're coming from ..."' She is in hospital because of the voices, which she is told are coming from her own head, but to Maggie that is 'a crock of shit. I think they're witches. I think they're using supernatural powers from far away to hurt me.' She knows that the voices are bad for her and that she must rid herself of them, but she believes that will never happen unless she is helped by people who share her view of them.

> I'd like to relate to people. I mean I'd really like to relate to someone who can understand me, my interests and my problems. If I had someone to be with twenty-four hours a day that would probably cure me. I mean if I had somebody with me all the time without leaving me I'm sure the voices would go away completely.

Few psychiatrists would take this prediction at face value, yet there are elements of it that are worthy of serious attention. For one thing, supportive relationships are known to have particular therapeutic value for people like Maggie. For another, psychiatrists have long speculated that an illness like Maggie's might have a different course if she were among people who to some extent saw things her way. She says, 'I'm into sorcery ... er ... religion ...' Undoubtedly she would still be suffering, and would still seem abnormal, even among others who were also 'into' sorcery and other non-mainstream religious ideas. But they would not flatly deny the reality of her witches, her voices. Perhaps she could be right in thinking that such people would have a different sort of access to her, and to her illness.

Nevertheless, most of the psychotics in New York would be lucky to be in Maggie's shoes. She is in a superb treatment facility, and she has the sturdy support of her sister and brother-in-law – in fact, they are part of her ticket of admission to the facility. In Jack Gorman's harsh calculus of healing, he wisely refuses to spend tens of thousands of dollars' worth of medical resources on patients whose situation out of hospital is so bad that their hard-won stabilization will not last even a few months. Impoverished, homeless, threatened, abused, constantly tempted to go off their prescribed medicines and substitute street drugs, drifting in and out of touch with the people taking care of them – these are the forgotten ranks of the mentally ill, cut off from the mainstream of life almost as much as they were when institutionalized.

Scores, if not hundreds, of them can be found a short way from Gorman's ultra-modern unit, using some of the thousand beds in the Armory. Here, in a vast single room, each inhabitant is allotted an eight by eight foot space to unshoulder some physical burdens and sleep. All are men; sometimes up to eighty per cent are black. They are the overall responsibility of the 'Super', a sort of overseer who represents City Hall, but the schizophrenics and manic-depressives among them are the burden of the medical superintendent, Doctor Alan Felix, and he takes this burden seriously:

> I think that having an understanding of what the relationship consists of and what your reactions are to the patient is vital. Sometimes the whole treatment will hinge on that, because if you are angry, do something that's punitive, or withholding, then you can lose that patient. And then all the Thorazine in the world won't help because you don't have a patient.

It is in the nature of schizophrenia that patients are cut off by the illness from normal social and emotional ties to others, so social support must figure in any treatment. Expecting medicines to do the job alone is like expecting aspirin or steroids to heal a broken leg, without ever setting it in a cast and without ever using exercise or physical therapy.

Taking care of these poor, homeless, extremely ill people in the

Armory, without even a fraction of the resources Doctor Gorman has just across the street, may not be a fool's errand, but it is certainly an uphill fight. Denis, for example, is a young schizophrenic who used to smoke purified cocaine – in his case almost a sure way to bring on a psychotic episode. By his own account he once defecated on himself, and he didn't care about what he looked or smelled like. Where one eye was missing he had a closed, sunken eye socket, without an artificial eye or a patch. His appearance speaks volumes about his social ties – or rather, lack of them; there was simply no one who had enough of a relationship with him to make him want to care how he looked. It was all he could do to control himself in the terrifying presence of the voices that constantly broke into his consciousness, telling him to kill himself and others.

Even in the bleakness of the Armory, with Doctor Felix's super-intendence, he has learned to care more. But the environment among such desperate men is dangerous:

> It is a frightening experience, because you don't know if they have any idea that you have money on you, and you get hurt seriously. They ... they pick out the ones that they think are the weakest, and they will attack them. They will take their food and whatnot. I have one eye, and a lot of people would get over on me because I do have one eye, and take my milk off my tray or take my food because I can't ... they know which side to do it on because I was wearing a patch at that time.

During a stay at Manhattan's Bellevue Hospital, Denis was able to get a glass eye, regain some of his physical strength and gain the upper hand over the voices for a time. Then he was able to go out again to the Armory and, with the help of Doctor Felix, have a chance of some further stability.

Homeless, mentally ill women in New York are even more vul-nerable, but the shelters are smaller and some of them at least appear to be safer. Florence, one of the residents at the shelter at 350 Lafayette, is grateful:

> I heard stories about shelters, that they beat up women, they ... they rob you, they molest you and stuff like that, and basically I was petrified. But I had faith in God, so I went to the shelter and from 85 Lexington they transferred me here to 350, and I felt very comfortable here, it's like home. Nobody bothers you, it's like a

family here, and it's ... it helped my mentality. Helps me, keeps me strong – it makes me focus on what I gotta do with myself.

She also calls it 'a place just to rest my head', doubtless meaning a lot more than what others usually mean by those words. She likens her medication to the insulin a diabetic must take, a compelling analogy that highlights the enormous, life-saving importance of psychiatric drug maintenance. Clearly Florence is getting some of the social support she needs so badly at this shelter.

Another woman at '350' points out, however, that this is no normal social network:

> You know, sometimes you feel, like, isolation. I got kids, and it's very hard because ... there are times I ... I got there on a Saturday, and my son says to me, 'Mommy, when you gonna come home, when you gonna get an apartment for us?' So I'm like, I'm like playing a big hero to him, and it's like I can't break his heart. I can't just say to him, Well, I'm in a shelter now and I can't take you with me. But I do tell them that I am sick, I am trying to get myself together, they're giving me medicine to, so I go see a doctor and everything and it's, One day I'll get an apartment for all of us and, you know, have faith with me, you know, take care, you know, don't worry – I still love you ...
>
> When I leave my son, I see, like, tears come out of his eyes, and he says 'Mommy, you gotta go now,' and I say yes I have to go, and I – it's hard to say goodbye to them, you know, it's like, O gee I wish I hadn't to go through this, you know, you be like O God, here I go again ... it's very hard.

Both these women talk about faith, but no ministry beside the psychiatric one seems to play a role in their care. After centuries in which the care of sufferers like them was almost entirely in religious hands, the absence of people who can help turn their faith to healing advantage is distressing. When working in psychiatric hospitals during my medical education, one of my most frequent questions was, where are the chaplains? One would think that theirs would potentially be one of the most powerful ways to reach people who are, after all, spiritually troubled by almost any definition, yet among the mentally ill poor, one sees few examples of religious ministry, whether explicit or indirect.

But this is not true everywhere, not even in New York. Near the St Francis monastery there is a welfare hotel that, like all such places for the poor, includes many who are mentally ill. Two members of the order chose to devote themselves to the medical, social and spiritual care of these lost, needy people. Father John McVane, one of the men, thought back to the dramatic changes of the 1970s, when he began the work.

> I stumbled into this privately owned [welfare] hotel near our monastery – and it turned out that this building was *filled* with people who had been what we now call deinstitutionalized. I don't know if the word even existed back then, but these were people who had been stabilized on these new medications, and it was felt that they could be released back to the community. Unfortunately there was no community. There was no family, no support system that would see that they would take the medications. Consequently they would get sick again, go back in the hospital, restabilize, back out, go off the medications, go back in the hospital. So what I stumbled upon back in the early seventies, as a social problem, was not homelessness, but something called the 'revolving door syndrome'. In fact what we created was a surrogate family, a surrogate community for these folks who didn't have a community – to provide the services that would enable them to stay out of the hospital.

The extent to which this community really serves as a family is indicated by the fact that when one of the residents dies, it is often the Franciscan brothers who arrange for the burial; there is frequently no one else to do it. Unfortunately most of the mentally ill poor in New York do not have even a surrogate community, much less a real one. Men like Father McVane or Doctor Felix, who are prepared to give a large part of their lives to provide desperately needed continuity of care for people with no other hope are few and far between.

To blame psychiatrists and other doctors for not solving the problem is to insist on the pretence of medical omnipotence and avoid taking on what is the responsibility of all of us. The doctors have been clear in telling us: their resources are exhausted long before their patients' needs have even begun to be met. They are clear in telling us, too, that there is no magic bullet for schizophrenia or any other psychosis; with all the drugs we have, the most that can be done is partly to stabilize a person who, with the right support from a community that cares, can stay stabilized for a lengthy period, and without that community, can't. Pixie, a Haitian mother now living on the street without her children, stares at the desolation around her and says, 'You see the skeletons of buildings, you see the skeletons of people, and . . .

it's a damn shame, *tu comprends?* You know – politics sucks.' Politics, not medicine; society, not doctors; *us*, not *them*.

Some people blame New York for having one of the worst problems of this kind, but in fact the streets there overflow with the homeless mentally ill precisely because New York has offered more – more welfare, more shelters, more free psychiatric care – than most of the rest of America. So the city becomes a magnet for people who have nowhere else to go, whose home towns and states have abandoned them, and is blamed, in effect, for even *trying* to take care of them.

And why are they ignored and neglected? Because the homeless mentally ill have no political voice; they cannot, by the nature of their problems and circumstances, form an effective political action group. Because suburban home-owners do not want halfway houses anywhere near their children – or threatening their property values. Because we have trained ourselves in our busy working lives to stare right through their frightened and frightening faces framed in matted hair. Because they remind us far too insistently of how vulnerable we all are, and how inhumanely we too will be treated if and when we have the bad luck to falter.

India has the second largest, and one of the fastest-growing populations of any nation in the world, so it is no surprise that millions of its people are homeless and living on the streets of its cities. But if there is a shortage of homes, there is often no shortage of relatives. Eighty per cent of the population still live in villages structured around extended families. That means that most people who become mentally ill will feel alone only to the extent that the illness itself keeps them psychologically out of touch. If and as recovery occurs, a family and a community will usually be there – to respond, converse, support, touch, comfort – in short, to make recovering more worth doing. Maggie's poignant appeal for company – 'If I had someone to be with twenty-four hours a day . . .' – is harder to imagine for similar patients in India. Someone is usually there.

In the holy city of Benares, for example, on the banks of the Ganges, people make religious pilgrimages – as families – to bathe in the river's sacred water. Akbur Puri, one of the villages near Benares, draws such pilgrims from distant places; they come to seek the help of traditional healers. Whether the victim is Hindu or Muslim, the belief is that it may help to bathe in the Ganges or actually to eat some of the holy pages of the Koran, while also seeking Western-style treatment from Western-trained psychiatrists. Somatic, or biological, treatments are respected, so the families of patients may demand pills and even electric shock therapy – an approach that is particularly esteemed.

Few are willing, however, to forgo parallel or simultaneous spiritual treatment, and Akbur Puri is also dense with specialists of this kind. Indeed, the mental hospital and clinic are surrounded by a vast, crowded camping ground consisting of patients, their families, and traditional adepts and spiritual healers. Just as Maggie's Indian counterpart would rarely have to suffer externally imposed isolation from other people, she would not have to look far to find many who would take her voices, her demons, very seriously. They would not be different in wanting to try to help her get rid of them, but they would set about doing so as believers, and thus as full allies of the patient against the spirit world, rather than talking down to her about nonexistent voices.

But perhaps most essentially, the social network that the Franciscan friars in New York had to build up so laboriously from scratch is already in place in Benares. Patients normally come for treatment with their families, who stay nearby, participate in consultations with the doctors, take full responsibility for helping with the treatment and above all provide a home and family for the patient to be discharged to – something that psychiatrists who care for the mentally ill poor of Manhattan often have no chance of finding for their patients.

An Indian psychiatrist, Doctor Indira Sharma, head of the Department of Psychiatry at Benares Hindu University, talks about one of her patients in terms any Western physician would understand:

> This lady is suffering from schizophrenia of one-year duration. There is a family history of a similar illness in her father as well. And it is nice that I find that the husband and the mother of the patient have also come in with the patient, and they also have expressed their keenness to cooperate in the treatment programme. I am advising her to continue these drugs for about two weeks, and then she can come in for follow-up. She has also been told that the drug treatment is very essential and how the family should deal with her when she is at home. And in particular they must not react strongly when she is not able to do her routine duties, for example the domestic duties which she is expected to do. They should not express their resentment. Rather they should be neutral and try to explain to her in a sympathetic way that she is ill, and we do not mind if she is not able to do her work, which she would certainly be able to do when she gets well.

These are the sort of understanding guidelines that Jack Gorman is able to give his patients and their relatives in the ward at Columbia, and that Alan Felix is unable to do at the Armoury where the mentally ill have no families to turn to, or any other support system.

Doctor Sharma also advises the patient and the family to stay away from alternative spiritual or Koranic healers, although that part of the advice is not likely to be followed. If the patient and family can faithfully apply all that they are told about drug management, social support and responsiveness, and return to the clinic for follow-up, then it may even be helpful to consult a spiritual healer as well. The doctor-patient relationship is well known to be a powerful aid in healing, especially in psychiatry. If the alternative healer can enter the symbolic world of the psychotic person, and converse about the psychotic thoughts in a serious, accepting way, the opportunity may therefore present itself for drawing the patient out of mental and emotional isolation.

As pointed out by one of Maggie's psychiatrists in Manhattan, she would still seem psychotic in a culture that believed, as she does, in witches, for other people would experience the witches in more predictable, controllable ways. Psychosis would not evaporate in a world where everyone has beliefs that a Westerner might call delusions, but a culture that is more open to these strange ideas might be able to meet the patient halfway. Or to put it another way, the support network around such a patient might consist not only of loving, concerned, well-prepared family and friends, but also of powerful symbols, language and meaning.

Perhaps the closest we have come to this in Western culture is to have taken seriously some of the images drawn, painted and sculpted by those among the mentally ill who have artistic talent. Vincent Van Gogh may be the most famous of these, but there are many others whose work contains images that have universal meaning but may only be generated by those who are steeped in the pain of psychosis. At a more straightforward level, however, visions like Van Gogh's *The Hospital at Arles* may be taken as depictions of the bleakness of mental hospital life. As John MacGregor, author of *The Discovery of the Art of the Insane* (1989), says, 'To value insights derived from psychotic experience is not to indulge in uncritical enthusiasm for insanity' – or, indeed, any enthusiasm at all. It is certainly not for us to say that the pain of the mentally ill is worth the visions they may have. But simply by paying attention to those visions, we may get a little closer to Maggie's dream of having someone to keep her company in her pain.

Siena is a beautiful old Italian town, set in the hills of Tuscany. In July each year, the local people – plus hordes of tourists – descend on the glorious central piazza for a centuries-old ritualized madness called the Palio. In this spectacular horse race each of the town's ancient guilds fields a horse and rider for a no-holds-barred series of turns around the medieval square. Before the race, each horse is taken into church to be blessed, and the jockeys are guarded day and night, forbidden to speak to anyone. During the frantic race those same jockeys flog each other with whips in the form of phalluses, and violence, among the crowd as well as the riders, is not unusual. The winner sucks a dummy and drinks milk and wine; the loser purges his digestive system by drinking castor oil.

It seems crazy. Yet in the realm of real craziness – the disordered thought and action of schizophrenics – Siena is much less of a mad race than New York, and devoid of the violence that psychotic people in Manhattan fear every day. Indeed the mentally ill of this ancient Italian town are neither figuratively nor actually the focus of the crowd: in the more relaxed culture of the Mediterranean world, they fit more easily, they do not have to prove their worth, their right to exist, every day of their lives.

Nevertheless, until recently Siena's mental hospital, San Niccolo – originally run by Franciscan friars – earned the quotation from Dante's *Inferno* emblazoned over its fourteenth-century arch: Leave all hope behind, you who enter here. Although from the time of Napoleon's conquests the hospital was officially run on rational principles, not devil-and-demon talk, it was in fact a living hell for most patients until the 1970s. Hundreds were in chains, many in solitary confinement; strong nurses and orderlies wrestled them into some sort of submission. Their terror and unremitting suffering were almost beyond belief.

Psychiatric theories put forward by Cesare Lombroso in the late nineteenth century dominated the twentieth: the mentally ill, like criminals, were born, not made, and society needed protection from them. In the time of Mussolini, these ideas fitted well with the Fascist mood. As elsewhere in Europe, and even in the United States, various strong measures to protect society, to set the mentally ill far apart, were deemed necessary. Oliver Wendell Holmes, the great American Supreme Court Justice, upheld a sterilization order saying, 'Three generations of imbeciles are enough.' H.G. Wells, G.B. Shaw and other leading intellectuals in Britain gave voice to similar ideas. For the Nazis it was not enough to sterilize them and set them apart; they went on systematically to murder them.

Then the anti-psychotic drugs came, to Siena as to almost everywhere else, and suddenly lives in the outside world were thinkable for these patients, sometimes after decades in chains. To ensure that the hospitals would not be tempted to hold on to their patients, Franca Basaglia, a Senator in the Parliament in Rome – who was married to a pioneering psychiatrist also involved in mental hospital reform – introduced a law that in 1978 codified the assumption that the state had no right to hold people against their will. The mental hospitals largely emptied, and practically overnight.

As in the United States, it was not an unreserved blessing. Doctor Livia D'Argenio, medical director of San Niccolo, has lived through both eras; she knows that problems apply to each:

> It isn't as easy as people think. I am in sympathy with many of the new reformers, but you cannot just let people go out into a vacuum. They have to go somewhere. All of the people here are free to go if they wish. In fact, the new law means that once they get outside, even if it's just for a visit to their friends, then they can't come back inside without a court order. It's rather a ridiculous state of affairs – the pendulum has swung too much in the other direction. The stigma of mental illness within our communities is still great.

Patients in hospital now are free to leave if they want to, but most of them don't. The hospital is their home, and with the medications available to them, it is not a bad one. But the world outside the hospital, for those less ill patients who can handle it, is far less forbidding than the corresponding world of the schizophrenic discharged into the bowels of New York.

This is illustrated by following the fortunes of a group of patients who had been residents in a Rome hospital, Santa Maria della Pieta, until 1988. Although the combined impact of the new medications and the Basaglia law should have given them their freedom years earlier, the hospital administration held on to them. Then one day an art therapist and another staff member took them for a day's outing to the country – and they never came back. They remained in Bracciano, the lakeside town, where the local general practitioner maintains them on medication and helps take care of them in other ways. The two dedicated and enterprising hospital staff members stay with them, using both government and private funds to look after them as outpatients – as free men and women.

When interviewed, the group had been out for a year, after being in Santa Maria for ten, twenty-five and in one case thirty-two years. One, Roberto, said that 'it was as if we had seen everything for the first time ... all at once ... and when we have had the opportunity to see beautiful things, we have felt a little ... it's as if certain things are asleep ... but they must wake up again.' Evonne Couvert, the art therapist, asks, 'And what are the beautiful things outside?' 'The beautiful things outside ... the nurse said, "If you are looking for peace, you will find peace ... when you are dead."' But has he found some peace here? 'Yes, I have found a little peace here ... of course, there are moments of sadness, but also good moments ... when you have a little more strength ... the body reacts better and the enthusiasms are ... let's say ... more satisfactory.'

'I like it here,' another man says. 'There is more peace. The lake keeps your personality calm ... it calms you down.' He had never liked having many people around, and in the hospital there had been too many people. With this group, he feels comfortable. Another man, Manuele, is asked what he had been looking for in the outside world. 'You mean the difference between here and there? Outside it feels great! We don't depend any more, all of us, on the hospital. Each of us has his own responsibility.'

At a town meeting in Bracciano, the mayor declares the incorporation of these mental patients into the town to be a source of pride. A physician, Doctor Sigillo, rises to say that 'this meeting should really fill us with joy, because the community is making a great effort towards the mentally ill people. And that means that an experiment, something new, has been carried out, conscientiously and with determination, to solve the problem.' He goes on to observe wisely that mental illness was born together with human beings, implying that it must be solved with human beings.

An older visiting physician, Professor Antonino Iaria, medical director of Santa Maria della Pieta, has waited a long time for this, at first unauthorized, experiment. 'I witness now with pleasure something that I have always maintained – that patients can leave the hospital, and they can do it well. I remember that in one of those meetings, in the year 1974–75, when we used to be angry, when I began talking about my plans, a nurse told me that I was an incurable optimist. I would like to tell the nurse now that my optimism had some results.'

Doctor Thommaso Losavio, also of Santa Maria della Pieta, expresses how important this experiment is now:

I don't think that it's enough to find a house where you can put people outside the psychiatric hospital, because that house itself can become a small asylum. It is important that this reality has its real location in the village, the borough where these people live, and that the community acknowledges this situation, not any more as strange, alien, but a reality which belongs to that community. If these people are recognized as citizens of this village, the village itself is transformed, because it becomes conscious of a reality which belongs to it, not imposed from outside, but a *suffering* which, in one way or another, exists in the village. The suffering itself is given a right of citizenship, and this allows the house not to be separated, excluded, but to be part of this context of life.

'The suffering itself is given a right of citizenship.' The words recall the dreams of Anne Waldschmidt and her friends in Bremen, Germany, dreams for the acceptance of disability as an integral part of human social life; and they recall Doctor Eric Cassell's warning that physicians must learn to deal with suffering as well as disease, or forfeit their right to be called healers. They are also a poignant reminder of the cry from that young mother living on the street in New York, staring around in despair at 'the skeletons of buildings, the skeletons of people', and then crawling back into the cardboard box that her 'community' has forced her to call home.

Doctor Arthur Kleinman has also thought a great deal about suffering. He has devoted his career to a single overriding idea: that the cultural and social context of illness, especially mental illness, is at least as important as any process going on in the body or brain. It is not that he does not believe in the power of those processes too, but that he has learned through decades of professional experience that in our time the emphasis on biological explanations of mental illness has once again gained ascendance. Millions of people in Western countries, most of them close to 'normal' – whatever that means – have found that they can tinker with their brain chemistry, not just with illicit but with safely prescribed drugs; and as a result they can adjust to lives that otherwise would be deeply unsatisfactory, by virtue of flaws that used to be thought of as philosophical or spiritual, not medical problems. People have come to terms with their lives by splashing drug cocktails – as well as the conventional kind – at their brains. Since not all human situations can be changed, this approach is not necessarily a bad thing. But by inference, the same people assume that those with more serious mental illnesses are basically medically ill, sufferers from brain disorders, full stop; and, by further inference, brain disorder must mean brain treatment.

As we have seen, however, few psychiatric illnesses, indeed few illnesses in general, can be legitimately dealt with just as biochemical problems. And Doctor Kleinman has been at the forefront in laying the foundations of a new kind of psychiatry that is a product neither of brain research laboratory nor psychotherapist's office, but is a broader, more enlightened discipline which can set those valid approaches to work in a real-world human context.

Kleinman is a psychiatrist who for decades has had daily responsibility for mental patients, including many of the most seriously ill and the most desperately poor. But he is also an anthropologist with years of experience in developing countries, among people whose ways of life and belief are so unfamiliar that they would baffle most Westerners. Although he uses the full spectrum of drug treatments, when he looks at a patient his vision extends far beyond the chemical slush of the brain and body, far beyond the walls of the consulting room, to a whole world of forces as uncomprehended by many psychiatrists as the space-time continuum was by physicists at the dawn of the twentieth century.

These are the social and cultural forces that help cause mental illness and that can worsen it or, with the help of medications and psychotherapy, turn it back towards health. They are as various as the stresses of homelessness and poverty, the humiliations of bigotry, the strength of religious faith, the isolation of loss and grief, and the fear of devils and demons. They can be as seemingly trivial as the contemptuous glance of a policeman, the backfire of a passing bus that reminds a man of war, or the trapped feeling a woman gets when her boss makes sexual jokes at her expense. They can be as charged as a father's rape of his child or the touch of a brother's loving hand on his sister's troubled brow. And they can be as exotic as the belief that eating pages of the Koran is curative or that a passing shadow is devastatingly harmful.

That these forces play an important role in illness is undeniable, for, much as we now know about genetic determination, it has repeatedly been proved that genes cannot explain all of mental illness. For example, a number of studies of identical twins in which one member of the pair has schizophrenia have found that the other twin has the same disorder only about half the time, give or take ten or fifteen per cent, depending on the study. This is a paradox for the theorist who looks only to biochemistry for explanations, because although it means that the genes are very powerful, it also suggests that the environment is about equally powerful. While some of this environmental effect is due to obvious physical trauma, like head injury and brain viruses, much of it cannot be simply explained and has to be due to the social and cultural forces that, after a century of psychiatric science, we still know very little about.

Hundreds of studies have, however, taught us a little more about what helps schizophrenics get better, and what helps keep them that way. There is no longer any doubt, even in the minds of the most biologically oriented psychiatrists, that patterns of culture and social life within the mental institution systematically influence the time it takes an acutely ill schizophrenic to recover enough to be discharged. It is equally well established that the pattern of interaction in a family, or in any group to which the improved patient is discharged, affects the likelihood and timing of a further breakdown; and that family therapy and an effective support network can significantly postpone, of not avoid, breakdown, even without change in the medications.

Clearly, the pleasant, friendly byways of the lakeside town of Bracciano will have a positive therapeutic effect compared to the empty urban canyons of New York, and even within Manhattan the hotel run by the friars will help keep schizophrenics well far better than the Armoury. By extension, it seems possible that cultures with strong family traditions and broad kin ties will be better places in which to be mentally ill than cultures in which the family has been worn down to a skeleton. This possibility is certainly suggested by what was seen in India, although proving it is something else again.

The concept that psychotic patients in the developing world recover more readily than those in the industrialized world has been discussed for at least half a century, but the evidence put forward is full of problems. First and foremost is the problem of diagnosis. As recently as the early 1970s, studies showed that British and American psychiatrists differed widely on the diagnosis of the same psychotic patients, with the Americans classifying most of them as schizophrenic while the British labelled them manic depressive. This was not a merely semantic dispute, since the label 'schizophrenic' led to treatment mainly with anti-psychotic drugs like chlorpromazine, while the 'manic depressive' label meant the patient might be stabilized on lithium, a drug with much rarer serious side-effects, and not often used in the US at the time. And the situation revealed some fundamental problems with psychiatric diagnosis: if two countries sharing the same language and similar cultures, even similar medical traditions, could be so different in their ways of categorizing psychotic people, what could be expected of comparisons between psychotics from very different cultures?

American psychiatrists moved in the direction of the British in diagnosis during the 1970s and 1980s, and lithium proved useful for more and more of their patients. But this did not overcome another crucial difference affecting comparative studies. Since the nineteenth century schizophrenia has been viewed as a basically chronic disorder, one that is likely to stay the same or get worse as the patient goes through life, while manic depressive illness has been viewed as a naturally cyclical one where periods of madness alternate with periods of relative mental health. Thus, if the chronic disease in question (schizophrenia) is often confused with a naturally cyclical one (manic depression), only the most rigorously controlled studies could convincingly show that recovery is faster and better in less developed countries. But decades of studies of the hypothesis lacked such controls.

Doctor Kleinman, together with his colleague Keh-Ming Lin of the UCLA Medical Center, recently reviewed this disappointing record and concluded that most of the studies of the hypothesis do not provide sufficiently good evidence that it is true. There are too many uncertainties about patterns of diagnosis in all the different countries and cultures being compared. There is also another serious problem. Schizophrenia can result in such disordered behaviour that, as we saw in New York, survival itself is threatened. A person suffering the same level of impairment in an underdeveloped country, where poverty, hunger and grim living conditions are widespread, may well not survive long. The psychiatrically sickest patients may thus simply not be around to be studied by researchers looking at how well they recover, and the result may be an over-representation in developing countries in favour of patients who are less impaired to begin with, and so more likely to recover in any case.

Lin and Kleinman are aware of all these problems, but are optimistic about the possibility that two major international studies conducted by the World Health Organization – one recently completed and one still in progress – may help solve them. Unfortunately, some major questions remain. The completed study followed 1200 patients in cities in nine countries: Aarhus, Denmark; Agra, India; Cali, Colombia; Ibadan, Nigeria; London, UK; Moscow, Russia; Prague, Czechoslovakia; Taipei, Taiwan; and Washington DC, USA. Of the total number of patients in the study, over 800 were classified as schizophrenic.

Two and five years later, the industrialized countries did have lower recovery rates on average, but recovery varied much more *among* the industrialized countries themselves, and also among the non-industrial countries, than it differed *between* the two types of countries. In addition, some of the centres had high rates of drop-out from their study samples. Finally, many of the 'schizophrenics' in India, Colombia, Nigeria and Russia had later to be re-diagnosed as manic depressives or other varieties of psychosis with better intrinsic prospects for recovery than true schizophrenics have. Lin and Kleinman believe that forthcoming results from the second international study being conducted by WHO will provide stronger support for the cross-cultural hypothesis of recovery, but that remains to be seen.

What is beyond question, however, is the need for humane treatment of the mentally ill. In Benares, India, there are simply not the resources to provide good treatment for the mentally ill poor, although their families are frequently there to provide a support network for recovery. In New York, in the incomparably richer USA, there is a similar lack of resources to provide decent treatment for the poor psychotic, who ironically might be better off in Benares than facing a lonely life in the bleakness of the Armory or on the unforgiving streets. Italy, for all its imperfections, is grappling bravely with the problems, and one psychiatrist at the meeting in Bracciano pointed to an underlying truth:

> Madness is a phenomenon universally recognized, but people's attitude towards folly changes, historically and geographically. And the attitude is often based on prejudice. Prejudice is basically fear of madness. Madness ... upsets people profoundly ... It causes in ourselves the worry that our own folly can be awakened.

But as Arthur Kleinman points out in his book *Rethinking Psychiatry*, there is another kind of prejudice, one that is pervasive in his own medical specialty, and one that he has spent his life trying to change:

> Cross-cultural comparison, appropriately applied, can challenge the hubris in bureaucratically motivated attempts to medicalize the human condition. It can make us sensitive to the potential abuses of psychiatric labels. It encourages humility in the face of alternative cultural formulations of the same problems, which are viewed not as evidence of the ignorance of laymen, but as distinctive modes of thinking about life's problems ... Most experienced psychiatrists learn to struggle to translate diagnostic categories into human terms so that they do not dehumanize their patients or themselves ... Irony, paradox, ambiguity, drama, tragedy, humour – these are the elemental conditions of humanity that should humble even master diagnosticians.

Irony, paradox, ambiguity, drama, tragedy, humour – they may be the elemental conditions of humanity, but they still do not come to our minds when we confront the mentally ill. Rather, we slap a medical label on them and confidently send them away. To be truly humane means to rise above our fears and accept the fact that the mentally ill, like the physically ill, are not so different from us that we could not be in their shoes. It means that one way or another we have to grant citizenship to suffering.

CHAPTER 7

LIFE

SUPPORT

T he senior citizen is a new man in Florida! my Uncle Herman announced one day in his broad Brooklyn accent, slapping me on the back with a big, healthy hand. 'You ought to come down there and study them!' It was around 1970; he and my aunt had moved a few years earlier to a South Florida community called Century Village. There are now many of these communities, each consisting of hundreds or thousands of small, mass-produced houses owned by retired couples or individuals – mostly women, given the higher death rates of men. There are accessible clubhouses bustling with activity – card games, theatrical events, political meetings, dancing – square, folk and ballroom – swimming, softball teams, bowling leagues. Nearby there are golf courses, affordable restaurants, markets and the ubiquitous shopping malls. Everywhere there are vigorous, cheerful people, ranging in age from the late fifties to the nineties, glad to be alive.

My conversation with my uncle was at the beginning of a vast cultural change in the United States that has taken a large and increasing minority of elderly people out of the areas where they spent their lives, away from their grown children and their grandchildren, and into communities filled with others like themselves. This movement was engineered by the senior citizens themselves. No one put them away in what some might see as remote ghettos. They decided to segregate themselves.

Sun City, Arizona, is one remarkable example of such a community. A new town built for exactly this purpose, its citizens – Sun Citians, they call themselves – swear by it. They allow grandchildren to visit only a few weeks a year, and no one under fifty-five may live there. 'Dutch' Schultz, a man in his mid-seventies, is one of the town's many amateur performers; decked out in a cowboy hat and string tie, he strums his guitar and sings the unofficial anthem to an audience of other septuagenarians:

> Sun City, USA,
> It's so outstanding in every way,
> It's great in the West and we're here to stay
> In Sun City, USA.

In the song, which Dutch wrote himself, he calls Sun City a 'heaven on earth' and praises its founder for giving it 'a heart to withstand the passage of time'. It ends, significantly, on the line, 'Sun City will never grow old.'

Later, Dutch and his wife Dee, a dancer who does routines that might daunt a person half a century younger, glide around an artificial lake on their boat and talk about life, death and dancing. 'Well,' Dutch says with a smile, 'the goal of all the activity [here] is to enjoy the rest of your life, whatever your aim is.'

> And we enjoy dancing, my wife and I . . . we teach dancing. I think Sun City people come out here to retire, but once they get here, they just feel a lot younger by seeing the activities that's going on, and – I don't know, it's just that young breeds youngness, the thought, the thinking of it. One thing just leads to another and first thing you know everybody's acting that way. My son, who didn't know anything about Sun City, asked me when I moved out here, 'What are you movin' to Sun City for? You goin' out there to die?' And I says, 'Heavens no, I'm goin' out there to start livin'.'

Dee is at least as emphatic about her fellow citizens:

> They don't have time to think about dying. The only time you think about dying is when a funeral home calls you and asks you if you've had your will made out, or if you've got your funeral plans made out. And that's the only time you think about dying. You're so busy around here – you get up in the morning and you have swimming, you've got aerobics and dance lessons, and you don't have time to think about dying. You've got a hard time just to visit your friends, we're so busy!
>
> Oh sure, we go to church, and I sing in the choir. We have our

times with God, and our devotionals, and those are the times that –
no, sure we think about dying, but we don't dwell on it. We have a
lot of fun out here in Sun City, and we ... we *love life*.

But just because Sun Citians don't like to think about dying doesn't
of course mean they don't die. And before they die most of them, as
doctors sometimes put it, 'try to die' – that is, they become critically
ill. Harold Chinlund, an eighty-two-year-old retired accountant, was
trying to die one day in 1991 when his wife brought him into Sun
City's Walter O. Boswell Memorial Hospital. As both of them knew,
he was suffering from a fatal disease, pancreatic cancer, but they had
been told he would have perhaps a few good months of life before
becoming very ill and dying from the tumour. Now pneumonia
superimposed on the cancer was threatening to rob him of the remaining promised months – months of golf, bridge, even bowling, and of
time to really say goodbye to his wife.

Mrs Chinlund is candid about their lack of preparation:

> I'm very ignorant in medical things. And when the two doctors stood
> there and said this is the only thing we can do to save his life at this
> point, I said, Well, you should do that. But I don't know what trauma
> he's going to be going through. Because I know so little about these
> things. And I think it's a shame that the public doesn't know what
> people have to go through to get well. Of course he won't ever be
> well, but they said that he would have at least three months relatively
> free of pain, and then they would start some other things on him.

But she continues in a vein that is more revealing:

> Harold and I never spoke about what would happen if we got in a
> situation like this. He seemed to think he was going to live for ever.
> And he didn't want to talk about it. In fact he wouldn't even tell me
> what he wanted to do in case he did die – whether he wanted
> cremation, or anything. He just would not talk about it. I didn't
> know what I should do. But I talked it over with the doctors, and
> they seem to think there is a little hope of getting him through this
> pneumonia ... if the cancer hasn't spread to his lower lungs. At the
> time of the operation ten days ago it hadn't spread any place but the
> pancreas – which *is* fatal, I know that. Cancer of the pancreas is fatal.
> But according to these doctors, they can't tell how long he might
> live.

Not long ago in medicine, pneumonia used to be called 'the old man's friend'. If Harold were to succumb to it this time, he might indeed lose the potential good months, but he would also be spared months of battling an extremely painful illness, punctuated by debilitating treatments, that would inevitably follow that time. Certainly, it is impossible to predict exactly how many months he might live – nothing in biology is totally precise – but he might also, as now seemed likely, have very little time. With pancreatic cancer, the ending is never in dispute, only the timing – and there is little leeway in that.

Harold's adopted daughter Kate, who arrives some days later, is a critical care nurse herself, and she regrets that aggressive treatment of the pneumonia has begun.

I've been working in the medical profession long enough to know that the outcomes of this stuff are predictable and fairly ugly. But if you're given a chance, why not take it – I can't fault him for doing that. I wish they hadn't done what they did – put him on a ventilator. I don't think he would have wanted that. And I love the man dearly. He's a really great guy. But I don't want him to be in pain, and I don't want him to be confused, and out of control ... And he currently is tied down, and can't talk, and doesn't really know what's going on, I hope. And that's not my dad, that's not what his whole life has been about. And I really hate to see it.

I honestly don't think that this 'treatment' is going to make my dad any better. And I don't think that he's going to have any comfort in the rest of whatever life he has left, and I feel very badly that it happened. Just because we *can* do it doesn't mean we should. Technology isn't always the greatest boon to everyone.

And the doctors have a lot of trouble with that, because they're doctors – they're supposed to *cure* people. And it's very difficult for a lot of the ones that I know to say, 'Gee, I can't.' I think the medical profession needs to know that it's okay to die. We don't have to save everyone, just to make another two months on a life. You know, we can say, 'Gee, I've had a good life, I'm ready to go' – and do that.

She talks at length with her father's third wife, trying to help her prepare emotionally for a loss that, if it does not come in the next few days, will come in the next few months. Mrs Chinlund, however, knows some things her step-daughter may not know: 'I've seen lots of men with cancer enjoy their lives. In fact the president of our club just died of cancer, and he went up to the last week or two enjoying himself.' A little anger flares between them, because they have different vantage points, different goals.

A day or two later the treatment fails, even in its short-term goal of stabilizing Harold's lungs and giving him the three months. Hearing this, and the new tone in the doctor's voice, wife and step-daughter no longer have any disagreement. Mrs Chinlund has perhaps needed these few days to adjust to the end coming sooner than she had expected. But in any case there is now no will on anyone's part to continue mechanical breathing and – in a phrase used earlier by Kate – the plug is pulled.

On the same day Ellen Extract, another loving daughter facing a similar situation, waits with her mother as her father undergoes kidney surgery. The mother says, 'Everything seems to break down at a different time. One thing is improving and something else is falling apart. Now the liver is affected.' The daughter's frustration with medicine's fix-the-broken-part approach is painfully clear:

> It's very hard to talk with one doctor, because each doctor is a specialist, and we really are confident in his specialty. But if we talk to the kidney doctor, and he says, Fifteen years ago we could do nothing, look how great it is now! I mean I realize he's doing his job, and I appreciate it. But what about the lungs? What about the liver? He's a whole person! And that's where the dilemma comes in. Because my father wants to live as a whole person. I do feel that they're overly optimistic. I think that everyone looks at their piece of the body, and how that's gonna react to their treatment – which I guess is good . . .

She is obviously unsure about the best thing to do, but she does feel that her father is angry at both her mother and her. Unlike the Chinlund family, they have discussed how they would handle a situation like this: no prolongation of pointless pain. Ellen's mother is more blunt: 'I spoke to his sister last night. And I told her that I will not sign for anything else. He knows that I had promised him I would not do this, I would not put him on life support for the sake of science.' But since she is not sure that the situation is hopeless, and there is nothing new to sign for, life support continues.

Life expectancy is increasing in most of the world; in Western industrial countries it is in the mid-seventies for men and near eighty for women. But this statistic gives little indication of what is happening late in life, since it is an average of the life-spans of those who die in infancy through to those who make it past ninety. A more revealing figure would be the naturally occurring maximum human life-span: the age the average person can live to, given good health habits and good medical care. There is evidence of a number of people living to between 110 and 115 years of age, but this applies to very few people and seems to reflect luck as much as health. Reports of even greater longevity among some remote human populations, such as herders in the Caucasus Mountains, invariably evaporate on scientific investigation; for instance, it has been found in some cases that a man is using the birth date of a father or grandfather with the same name. Probably a figure in the nineties is about right for the average maximum human life span, although even this figure is a moving target. With good medical care, it can rise further.

More difficult to define in the elderly may be the meaning of disease itself. It used to be said that people died of old age, but people, however old they are, really only die of diseases. Cure the disease of a nonagenarian, and that person will leave the hospital just as surely as the cured thirty-five-year-old. Moreover, the quality of life in old age seems almost indefinitely improvable. Cataract surgery, hip replacement, pacemakers, hearing aids, false teeth, glasses, sleep aids, heart-beat-strengtheners and anti-depressant drugs go a long way towards undermining ancient truisms about old age. And if you have quality of life, then not surprisingly you want to keep extending it.

However defined, every year in every industrialized country there are more old people than there used to be, whether counted in absolute numbers or as a percentage of total population. Britain preceded the United States in this trend and is ahead in many ways in learning to deal with it. But there will be still more old people with each passing decade. At the beginning of the 1980s, when optimism about this development was still unreserved, James Fries, an authority on ageing, advanced a theory known as 'the rectangularization of the survivorship curve'. This mouthful of academese meant that no longer would a few per cent of people die at sixty-five, a few per cent more at sixty-six, and so on into the nineties – which in the past produced a long sloping graph of the number of people still surviving – but instead almost everyone would be living till, say, eighty-five, and dying in a great bunch by, say, age ninety. The survivors, if graphed, would show an almost horizontal line, sloping only slightly until age eighty-five, then making a precipitous vertical drop between eighty-five and ninety. In time the graph of survivors by age would approach the shape of a rectangle.

The same idea is expressed more vividly in a comic poem by Oliver

Wendell Holmes, the nineteenth-century American physician and author. In it a deacon frustrated by flaws in every carriage he has owned invents a 'wonderful one-hoss shay' ... 'that was built in such a logical way/It ran a hundred years to the day'.

> You see, of course, if you're not a dunce,
> That it fell to pieces all at once, –
> All at once, and nothing first, –
> Just as bubbles do when they burst.

According to this 'one-hoss shay' theory, future people with good health habits and medical care will not wear out one organ at a time, getting ill and staying ill for decades; instead they will stay healthy as they age, then suddenly all their organs will collapse simultaneously, according to a genetic plan for the bursting of the organismal bubble.

Unfortunately, although Fries still defends the idea, this does not seem to be the way things are going so far. As Edward Schneider, John Rowe and others have pointed out over the years since, there has instead been an increased variation in the age at death, persistent variation in the state of health at any given age, and a large subgroup of people who become ill early and stay ill for a long time as they age. At the same time the group over eighty-five has seen the fastest increase in numbers and the greatest decline in mortality. Most important of all, advances in medical research are making possible more and more interventions every year to treat the diseases of the very elderly. Those people – indeed everyone over sixty-five years of age – have health needs that are colossal, constantly increasing and, theoretically, given the march of science, infinitely expandable.

Daniel Callahan, Director of the Hastings Center in New York, a think-tank for biomedical ethics, has spoken out frequently on this problem; although not a physician, he is a respected authority on the health care needs of the ageing in the United States. As he wrote recently:

> In 1980 people over age sixty-five – eleven per cent of the population – accounted for twenty-nine per cent of the total American health-care expenditures of $219.4 billion. By 1986 the elderly accounted for thirty-one per cent of the total expenditures of $450 billion. Annual Medicare costs [the publicly paid portion of elderly health-care bills] are projected to rise from $75 billion in 1986 to $114 billion by the year 2000, and that is in current, not inflated,

dollars ... By the year 2040, it has been projected, the elderly will represent twenty-one per cent of the population and consume forty-five per cent of all health-care expenditures. How can costs of that magnitude be born?

The question seems rhetorical, but Callahan goes on at some length to show that they cannot – not without giving up many other things that we cherish, such as the health care of families with children or the education of the young.

For example, in 1986 a liver transplant, which a few years before was an experimental treatment reserved for young people in otherwise excellent shape, was given to a seventy-six-year-old woman in Pittsburgh. Since then articles have appeared in top US medical journals with titles like 'Open-Heart Surgery in Octogenarians' and 'Outcomes of Surgery in Patients Ninety Years of Age and Older'. And a 1991 report of the Institute of Medicine of the US National Academy of Sciences called for greatly increased investment in research on ageing and training of geriatric medical specialists. Clearly, costs for the medical care of the elderly and for the development of new technologies are open-ended.

The solution Callahan proposes is simple, radical, Draconian; we must, he believes, eventually establish a cut-off at a certain age – say, eighty – after which we will no longer *allow* major, high-expense medical and surgical interventions, even if they are life-saving. Callahan argues that people of such an age have already either lived full lives or had a reasonable chance to do so. They have had not only their biblical three score and ten, but ten more – a 'natural life span' – and consequently death for them would be a 'tolerable death'. To support this idea he cites the fact that people usually grieve in a different way after the death of an older person than after the death of a child or a young adult – one often described as untimely.

There seems to be some cross-cultural validity to these ideas. The Eskimo practice of setting old people off on an ice floe is often referred to, an act that seems to have been done with great reluctance, in the spirit of assisted suicide, not murder. And it was only done after giving the best care for the old that the Eskimo could afford, providing full physical and emotional support, with solicitous care during illness, and, above all perhaps, treating them with respect.

Similarly, among the !Kung San, or Bushmen with whom I lived in the Kalahari in Botswana, elderly people were traditionally treated with the greatest attention and respect – until their infirmities became a burden that threatened the survival of their children and grandchildren.

Then, and only as a last resort, an old person might separate from the rest of the group and quietly succumb to exposure and weakness in the familiar bush country where he or she had spent a lifetime. In contrast, the illness of one young mother led a healer to – as he described it – go to the world of the spirits to tell them in no uncertain terms that this person was too young to die.

But people like the Bushmen or the Eskimo – not very different in their ways of life and their options from our own remote ancestors – did not have the sort of death we often have today, which might be referred to as the long goodbye. Our death-defying technology, from cardiopulmonary resuscitation to the most powerful antibiotics, from blood-pressure-raising drugs to breathing machines, is able abruptly to stop someone from dying who has years of active life left to live. But it can also very often function to draw out the process of dying in a person whose time has really run out.

This problem can arise at any age – in the neonatal intensive care unit, for example – and the most celebrated cases have been about people neither at the beginning nor the end of life but in its undisputed prime. Karen Ann Quinlan was in her twenties when a car accident left her in a coma. A mechanical respirator was used to keep her alive: she had apparently lost function even in the most primitive part of her brain, which controls breathing, and had no function left in any higher part of her brain – the parts that enable us to feel happy or sad, to recognize our loved ones, to watch television and see more than a flickering light, even to know that time is passing. She was what is technically called 'brain dead'.

After seven months of this inhuman existence, her father went to court to obtain an order for the hospital to turn off the respirator. Counter-arguments held that this would be tantamount to murder. But the petitioners argued that Quinlan's life was being wrongly extended with a technology that could not have been considered by those who designed our traditional ethics. The respirator was not saving her life, merely abusing someone who was dying – or by some definitions, already dead. The New Jersey Supreme Court was persuaded by the petition, and the respirator was turned off, but Quinlan proved able to breathe by herself and did not die for another nine years. This was the first of many surprises and complications that would make these ethical issues much harder to tackle in reality than in the abstract. But the case provided an impetus to the notion that there might be a right to die, or at least, if one is dying in any case, a right to die unmolested by useless, even cruel, technology.

A more recent, equally celebrated case was that of Nancy Cruzan,

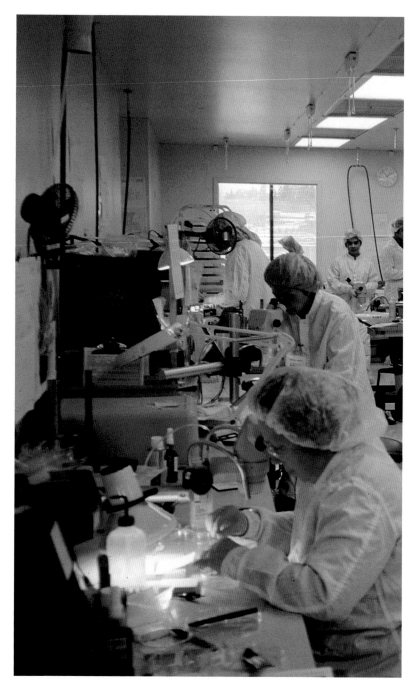

11 The rotoblator: the latest gizmo in cardiac surgery, manufactured at Heart Technology Inc., Seattle.

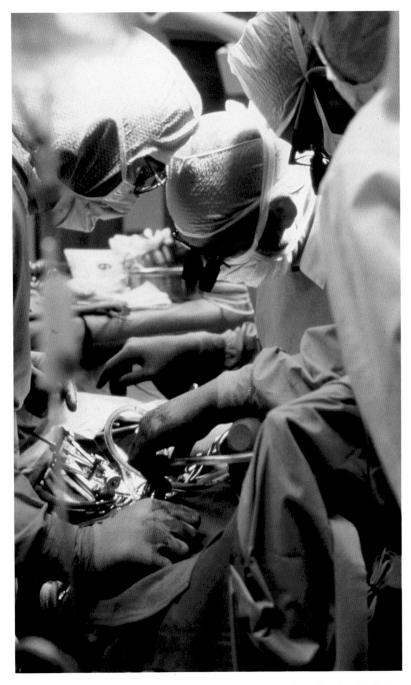

12   Dr Delos Cosgrove, chief of cardiac surgery at the Cleveland Clinic, Ohio; repeats of failed cardiac bypasses are the most common operation he performs.

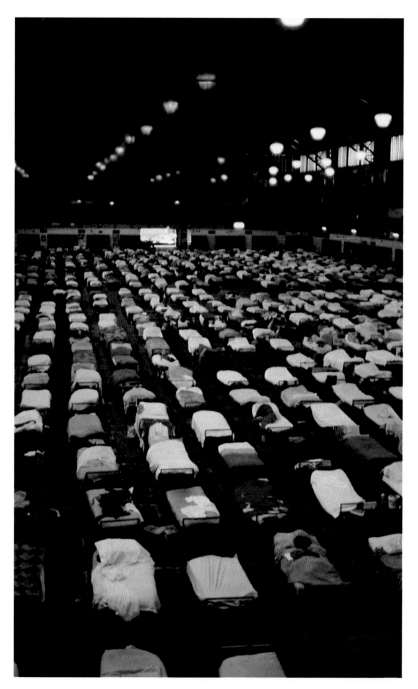

13　The Armory provides shelter for 800 homeless men in one room in New York City. Many are schizophrenic and manic depressive; the violence and fear they experience there work against recovery.

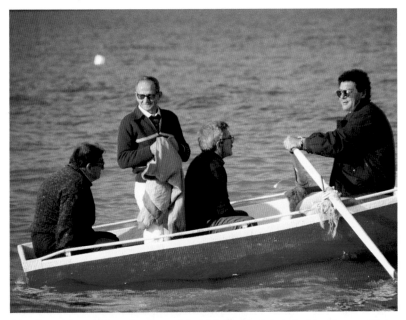

14 Ex-patients from the Santa Maria della Pietà hospital in Rome. They went on a day's outing with staff members to the lakeside town of Bracciano and never came back.

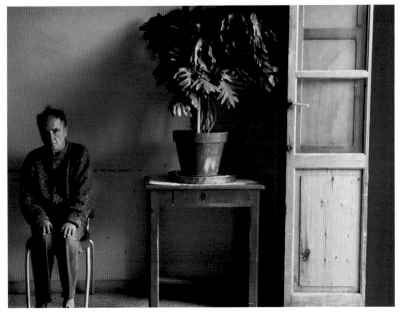

15 Waiting for lunch at the San Niccolò hospital in Siena; few patients remain in Italy's old-fashioned mental institutions.

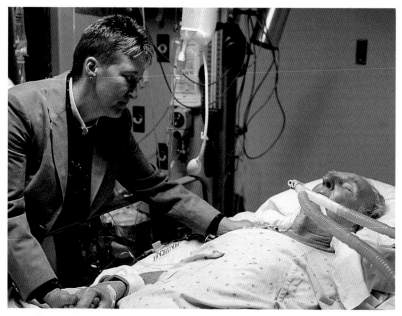

16   Sun City, Arizona. Harold Chinlund fights a post-operative pneumonial infection in Boswall hospital where he died a few days later; with him is his daughter Kate.

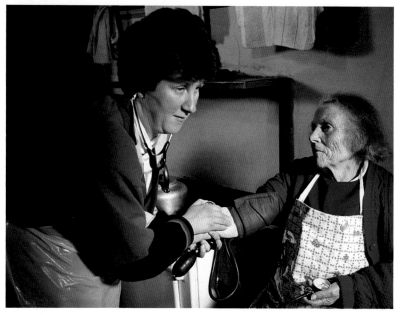

17   Public Health nurse Mary Syron is part of the community care team in Clifden, Co. Galway, in the Republic of Ireland, which helps elderly people like Abby Conneally to live independently at home.

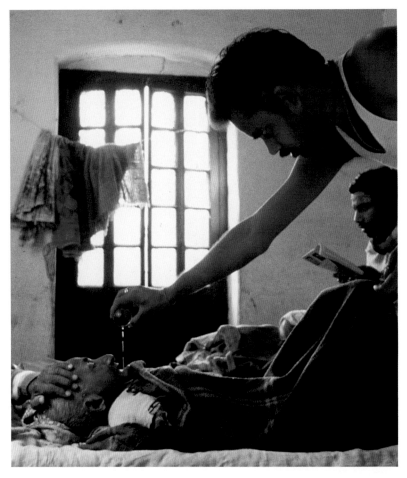

18   At the moment of death, water from the holy Ganges is trickled into the mouth of the dying.

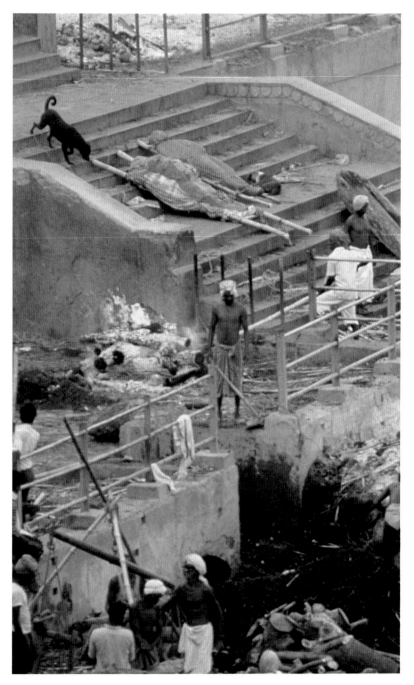

19   Bodies await their turn for cremation, having been given their 'last bath' in the Ganges.

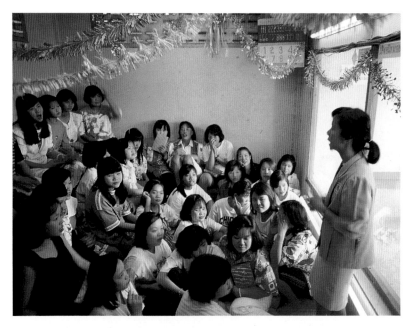

20   Teenage prostitutes in Chiang Rai, Thailand, having an urgently-needed sex education lesson.

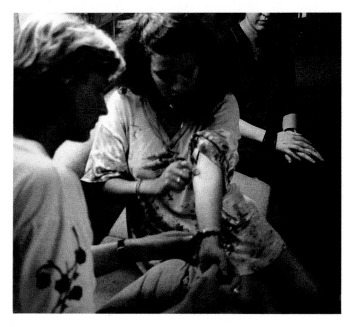

21   A street girl in Sydney receives a medical check in the AIDS Bus, by which doctors are bringing health education and treatment to the streets where it is most needed.

who finally died in 1991. At the age of twenty-five, in 1983, she had a car crash that caused severe brain damage, though not as severe as Quinlan's. She was not completely brain dead, could breathe by herself, and was not even thought to be dying, but she had to be fed through a feeding tube and unlike, say, a demented person who gets pleasure out of a teddy bear, or a quadriplegic who can't speak but who can enjoy the visits of relatives, she was unable to get anything whatsoever out of life. Yet she might live for thirty more years. Her distraught parents asked the courts to permit the feeding tube to be withdrawn, which would cause her to die of starvation. A lower court said yes, but the Missouri Supreme Court said no, citing the sanctity of life for their decision.

It was generally agreed that withdrawing food and water was not the same as turning off a mechanical ventilator. But the case ultimately turned on the issue of whether Cruzan's parents could show that she would have rejected all treatment, including the feeding tube, if she could have been asked in advance what she would have wanted. Although the US Supreme Court was not persuaded that this was so, the feeding tube was eventually removed. Since starvation and thirst are an unpleasant way to die, Cruzan was made as comfortable as possible with sedatives and pain-killers. Her parents stayed with her, and when she died they were relieved, yet also stricken with grief.

This and other cases had to do with the right of individuals to refuse treatment, or at most with the right of families to protect their loved ones from unwanted treatment. It was not considered relevant that Nancy Cruzan's care was costing the state of Missouri $130 000 a year and had already gone on for eight years. The courts did not ask what medical or other services were withheld from other people in need, in a world of limited resources. They decided that individuals have a right to die in certain circumstances, particularly if they have put their intentions in writing in what is called a 'living will' or, even better, if they have legally designated in advance someone to decide for them if and when they become incompetent. No such document as a living will is recognized in Britain, but preliminary discussions that could lead to a change in the law were under way in the House of Lords in 1992.

However the right to die by refusing treatment is different from a right to suicide, and a right to get assistance in suicide, particularly assistance from a physician, is something quite different again. The latter issue is under active discussion in many countries. In an article in *The New England Journal of Medicine* of March 1991 called 'The Physician's Responsibility Toward Hopelessly Ill Patients', twelve leading American physicians acknowledged that withdrawal of life support from such patients is quite common, that assistance in suicide is not rare and that many physicians have knowingly given a dying patient in great pain a dose of a narcotic or sedative high enough to hasten the end of life. All but two of them believed 'that it is not immoral for a physician to assist in the rational suicide of a terminally ill patient'.

In Britain two celebrated cases of apparent euthanasia have come to the courts. In each case a consultant was charged with attempted murder after allegedly administering a lethal injection of potassium chloride to a terminally ill patient. The first prosecution failed in 1990. In the second, the doctor was found guilty of attempted murder in September 1992, and was given a twelve-month prison sentence suspended for a year.

In parliament an all party committee, chaired by Lord Winstanley, a medical peer, has been sponsored by the Voluntary Euthanasia Society, a private organization, to consider issues relating to the right to die and euthanasia in British law. It is expected slowly to explore possibilities for legislation on these issues during the 1990s. The Society claims that around ninety MPs favour such legislation in some form but were reluctant to discuss it openly before the 1992 election. Opposition from the pro-life (anti-abortion) lobby is expected to be intense. Despite a 1985 poll that showed seventy-two per cent of the British public approving of active voluntary euthanasia, know-ledgeable observers believe that changing the law may take two or more parliaments because of the political complexities. Experience elsewhere suggests that practice will change before the law does.

In the Netherlands, such views have become very widespread among physicians as well as the public, and euthanasia, although it is strictly speaking against the law, is common. Doctor Carlos Gomez, an internist or general medical doctor who also has a PhD in policy studies, recently studied this Dutch practice on a case by case basis and published the results in 1991 in *Regulating Death*. His research raises doubts that in some cases tolerance of euthanasia is abused. Patients who request assistance in suicide may get a psychiatric evaluation, but treatment with anti-depressant drugs, for example, may be too brief to allow them a real chance of success. Nor are doctors dealing with terminal patients in pain always well skilled in pain management, and more effective pain control might in some cases postpone or remove their patients' desire to die.

Doctor Gomez also draws the line firmly where patients *demand* that a reluctant physician assist in suicide. Such demands have the potential to undermine gravely the physician's most important role – that of the patient's ally in battling disease and premature death. As he says in conclusion:

> The claim to a right to death at the hands of a physician is essentially a private claim on a public good ... a claim that I doubt can be justified ... Moreover, it needs to be shown how physicians can be allowed to kill at some patients' requests yet also be trusted not to kill when the temptation is there – either from the seeming hopelessness of the patient's condition, pressures from the family, or financial imperatives.

Daniel Callahan is equally opposed to euthanasia and physician-assisted suicide, but his notion of across-the-board withdrawal of major interventions after a certain age has met with a very unfriendly response from most doctors. Christine Cassel, John Rowe and Richard Besdine, among other leading American physicians who care for the elderly ill, have strongly criticized his proposal. Cassel, who is Chief of Medicine at the University of Chicago medical centre, calls it 'misleading and even dangerous', and points to a near-future probability of five million excess deaths as a result of it. While withholding treatment is very different from euthanasia, the plan is uncomfortably reminiscent of the early twentieth-century German medical treatise, *The Release and Destruction of Lives Devoid of Value*.

Yet the ice floe is not the gas chamber. Callahan argues that, far from resembling Nazi killing of Jews, gypsies, homosexuals and mental defectives, his plan would withhold treatment – not kill – in a completely non-discriminatory way, because all of us, regardless of race, colour, creed, sexual habits or mental status, equally accumulate years of life. Of course the rich octogenarians would still manage to get treatment one way or another, but he argues that no society can undertake to offer all its members every chance at life that the richest can afford. For example, no one has proposed that the National Health Service in Britain or Medicare in the US should fund private jet transport for poor heart patients to travel to the best transplant centres in the world.

Callahan's critics have been careful to separate his proposal from discussions of the right to die and the right to suicide, assisted or not. As Cassel writes, 'It is one thing to let people die because their lives have become an inconvenience to them; it is quite another to let them die because their lives have become an inconvenience to us.' Cassel believes that such a practice will wear through the moral fabric of our society and render us thick-skinned in relation to all kinds of wrongs. She also stresses the human cost of a blanket condemnation of the elderly to illness without intervention:

> Even if biological life-span is limited to ninety-five to one hundred years, there will easily be twenty million people over age eighty [in the US alone] by the year 2020. Most of them will be healthy, active people who could contribute to society if our society would allow them to do so. Treatment of a life-threatening illness in an eighty-five-year-old could save ten or fifteen years of life.

Noting that the elderly are the most diverse, least generalizable group in our society, she also says, 'The current ageing of society is an unprecedented event, a success of civilization . . . It is the challenge of our success that we create employment, educational and economic structures, and medical care that give all of us as we grow older a positive attitude about the future and about the people with whom we share our society.'

But even if we decide that we must make every reasonable effort to keep the old alive and well, we will still have to decide just where and how the health care budget for them should be spent. When William Miller, a Sun Citian, for example, came to the Sun City Hospital, he was drastically short of breath and accumulating life-threatening levels of fluid in his tissues. Like Mr Chinlund, Mr Miller had pneumonia; but unlike Mr Chinlund, he had no immediate life-threatening illness, so the pneumonia was not his friend. Had he gone to his doctor a few days earlier – or if, as in the old days in the US, his doctor had gone to him – he would not have come to the hospital, as Doctor Lauren Turley, the doctor who was on duty, puts it, already 'knocking on the door'.

> The social problems are more of an obstacle than the medical problems. Two patients live with each other, they barely are keeping each other in a living situation. One of them gets admitted, and then we immediately have a problem with the other one who can't stay alone by themselves. We have to deal with that a lot out here.

Mrs Miller, also ill and wheelchair-bound, could offer her husband no assistance, and Sun City's fragmented network of volunteers was inadequate to monitor or halt his downhill slide. Even the simple act of picking a patient up off the floor of his home must often be performed by paramedics – the first and only help to come to the scene.

But in Clifden, a beautiful old seaside town in the rolling Connemara countryside of County Galway, in the extreme west of Ireland, the social problems are handled rather differently. Although for generations the youth of the west of Ireland have emigrated, mostly to the United States, enough young people have stayed so that Clifden is hardly a town composed solely of senior citizens like Sun City. And far from limiting the visits of grandchildren, Clifden's elderly welcome their grown children living there and cherish their grandparent role. In the community hall people come together for musical evenings and dances in the same way that they have for generations.

The coming of old age may be no more enjoyable than it is in Sun City, or even less; but it carries with it complex rewards of status and place. The elderly have grown up here, have a sense of belonging, and they have a role to fill, caring, teaching and being models for the young. And as the infirmities of the last years of life creep up, they can more confidently expect the response of those around them to be one of affection and respect.

Ireland cannot afford the kind of 'heroic' hospital care that was given to Mr Chinlund and Mr Extract in Sun City, and Clifden's elderly may well not get that extra time granted by sophisticated medical technology. But if one thinks of the last events of those two men's lives in the Sun City Hospital as a kind of abuse of the elderly and dying, then Ireland's inability to match them might not seem so unfortunate, especially given the kind of medical care Clifden's elderly receive in the next-to-last phase of their lives.

The circumstances that led to William Miller's hospitalization would be quite unlikely in Clifden. He found himself getting increasingly short of breath; his wife, who had her own health problems, was in no position to monitor his health or to take him to the doctor. Several days passed and his breathing difficulties worsened. He still did not go to the doctor. Was it too difficult to get out and get over to the doctor's surgery? Was some mental weakness contributing to his self-neglect, or was it misplaced pride, or fear? Or perhaps he had the kind of medical insurance that required him to pay for visits to his doctor, but not for being rushed to the hospital in an emergency. In any case, he waited until his life-threatening shortness of breath resulted in an expensive hospitalization, not to mention needless anxiety and pain.

In Clifden, such a situation would probably have been prevented because of someone like Mary Coyne. She is a 'home help', a kind of visiting social worker; her job is to keep tabs on William Miller's Irish counterparts, the infirm elders of Clifden. A heavy-set, dark-haired woman, she talks about why she does the work she does:

> I was born and reared in this area, and as you can see it's a lovely, tranquil spot. I went away for a number of years, and I think coming back has taught me to appreciate it that much more. And having seen older people in different countries, and how they are cared for – a lot of it what I would call 'in' technology – here we still have sort of hands-on care, and the personal contact with the older people.

What she saw during her years in England did not impress her. Although there, too, home visits to the elderly and infirm are made by nurses and GPs, as part of the National Health Service, and home helps and other support workers may be provided, the level of service varies from one local authority to another, particularly with recent, increasing cut-backs in budgets. More importantly, as families have scattered, the elderly are often left isolated, and liable to impersonal care within a much changed community. Mary Coyne returned to the place she grew up in, where she felt she could help deliver a care more in accord with her values:

> I think older people need to be loved, to see that they are still part of the community, that they still have an input in that community, and that they won't be isolated – they will be allowed to live in their own homes, in their own communities, and virtually live and die in the communities that they were born in.

As part of her work now, she drives to the home of Bridget and John Conneely, a couple in their eighties whom she visits three times a week. She helps Bridget out of bed, gets her up and walking, helps a little in the kitchen, has tea with the two of them, chats about politics, and laughs with them – all at the expense of the taxpayers of Ireland.

It is money well spent. Coyne sees her role as 'mostly social', but at times it 'crosses over' and 'becomes medical' in the sense that she can monitor the health of people like Bridget and John, and, with the help of nurses and doctors who also make house calls, prevent deterioration that would lead to a disruptive and expensive hospitalization. Also, by running through simple domestic routines with them three times a week, she helps them to maintain skills that might otherwise be eroded and increase the risk of falls or other accidents that often devastate the lives and health of the elderly. *Use it or lose it* is a basic principle for the elderly, but even if they are physically incapacitated, a home visitor like Mary Coyne can help them retain their independence by both practical assistance and emotional support.

Bridget says that Mary is in a way better than a daughter. 'Because my daughter is away from me, but Mary's coming every second day to me, and that means a lot to me, doesn't it.' John concurs: 'She means a lot to me and a lot to Bridget as well. Because when she comes here three days a week she gets her out of bed and she washes her and changes her clothes and freshens her up and that's worth a lot to me – I'm not able to do all that.' By mobilizing Bridget and helping her to keep clean, Mary Coyne also helps to prevent bed sores and infections. By simply visiting and chatting with the two of them, she helps stave off the debilitating psychological depressions to which older people are easy prey.

Mary Coyne believes that her love for the elderly stems from her childhood, 'where my grandparents lived with us, and they were a second family, people we could go to for advice and love and an extra cuddle and sit on their knee for longer than we could my mother, because she was busy.' The culture of caring for the elderly of Clifden has thus perpetuated itself through a social structure in which family generations stayed together, something now much less common in many countries, and which Mary Coyne compares favourably to her experience in England. She feels that 'here in Ireland it is much more personal. And I can only speak for myself – that is the kind of care that I would want for my own family, and ultimately for myself when I am ... when I require help.'

For most of Clifden's senior citizens, home helps such as Mary Coyne are the most frequent official visitors, but there are also regular visits from a nurse and a doctor. Nurse Mary Syron makes calls once a week, which, under the Irish health system, as in the UK, are free; so too is any medicine the elderly may need. 'They are also entitled to equipment if need be,' the nurse explains, 'like a commode, a wheelchair or a walking frame.'

From what I can gather from my visit to America, there are no GPs who go out to the houses visiting people or who are called out to the houses; people have actually got to go to the hospital or to the emergency room to be seen. And there are probably no home helps provided by the government, or nurses working within the community. And health care is always a worry to people, that maybe they are not going to be able to afford it.

Mary Syron pointed to the vivid contrast with Ireland:

> Here if you have a medical card, and most older people do, then they
> can rest assured that they are going to have whatever visits they need
> from whatever member of the community care team without having
> to think, Well, am I going to be able to financially afford it? The
> older people in Ireland have entitlements that – say, if they're living
> alone they get an extra living-alone allowance. They have a fuel
> allowance just to make sure that they are adequately warm.

In short, the emphasis is on caring rather than curing. The strategy is
to spend small amounts of money on a regular basis to prevent health
crises, rather than to let things slide – put bluntly, to ignore people –
until such a crisis arises, and then to pull out all the stops to save the
life of a hospitalized patient, at a cost of thousands of pounds.

Doctors too play their roles in caring rather than curing. As the
home help visits three times a week and the nurse once a week, so
the local general practitioner makes a house call once a month. Doctor
John Casey – or Doctor John as he is affectionately known – readily
admits that Clifden is no Shangri-La. Because of the emigration of
able-bodied adults, the greater part of the population is made up of
the elderly and the very young – people with the greatest health needs.
In this situation the health care system must in some ways take the
place of the family.

He admits too that there are many things Irish medicine can't do
because of lack of 'resources, which are far greater in the States'. For
example, his patients must sometimes wait two or three years for a hip
replacement operation, one of the most successful operations in all of
surgery, giving crippled people their lives back. By the time an Irish
patient finally reaches the top of the waiting list, deterioration may
have gone too far in other ways for the procedure to bring full benefit,
besides the pain and disability suffered meanwhile. Long waiting lists
for non-urgent operations – where the issue is the quality of life rather
than the threat to life itself – can also be a problem in the UK. From
his experience as a general practitioner in Wales, Doctor Julian Tudor
Hart has argued that frugal Britain, in spite of its more technological orientation than Ireland, performs far too few coronary bypass
operations, leaving many of his patients – middle-aged and elderly
Welsh miners – on waiting lists, while years of their lives are spent in
pain.

On the whole, however, Doctor John much prefers the Irish system
to that in the States, where he spent part of his training and came away

deeply impressed by the differences in the way medicine is practised. Although he saw many exceptions, there is little doubt in his mind that American doctors are as a rule much more interested in money than Irish doctors are. And he is convinced that the result is a less caring kind of doctoring than is routinely practised in Ireland.

Despite all the arguments against overly aggressive treatment for the elderly – 'flogging' the patient is one slang word for it – physicians in Britain and the United States do not see themselves as prolonging life for no good reason. Doctor Farid Ghebleh, who is taking care of Harold Chinlund, the man with pneumonia on top of his pancreatic cancer, explains his thinking in these situations with the elderly:

> My personal philosophy is that we need to give them every chance that they have, we need to work hard to save their lives. We should be very practical and not philosophize too much when you're dealing with an individual patient. I've had frequent examples of people who really looked, like, dead – they looked like they had absolutely no chance, and they came back. They're more than anecdotal cases – in my past five, six years of critical care practice I've seen numerous of those cases.

He also feels that doctors should 'do everything until we have enough objective reasons to withdraw and stop that kind of therapy'.

In principle, this must be right. But on the phrase 'enough objective reasons to withdraw and stop', there hangs a long tale of cultural differences, scientific ambiguities, medical traditions and philosophies that differ not only among nations and religious groups but even among families and individuals. What would be a good death in Clifden might seem needless or even neglectful in Sun City. And what seems good and routine medical practice in Sun City might strike the Hindus of India as sacrilegious and the Irish as cruel – not to mention wasteful of precious resources. Sooner or later we have to recognize that those resources are not just pound or dollar signs ringing up in the eyes of health bureaucrats. The thousands spent trying to give Harold Chinlund three more months translate into services withheld from others. A dozen wheelchairs. A hundred visits from someone like Doctor John. A year of Mary Coyne's salary.

These are the kinds of services that would almost certainly have saved the life of Harold's neighbour William Miller, the man whose pneumonia had reached an unnecessary crisis. The best critical care that America had to offer was not up to the task of bringing him back from the edge, and he died a few days later – a death caused essentially by a *social* failure, and a death far more expensive than it would have been to prevent. Something is wrong, the people of Clifden would surely say, with the social and medical philosophy that surrounded Mr Miller's death – an untimely one for all his having lived past three score and ten.

Yet one of the main fears of elderly Americans is that they will not be allowed to die when the time comes, or even when the time has long passed. Members of the Hemlock Society in Sun City – an international group for the promotion of death with dignity, run by Derek Humphry, a Briton who was a distinguished journalist in England, then America – talk about their real experiences and their equally real fears.

A woman in her mid-sixties speaks through her tears, her voice breaking, about nursing her terminally ill brother in 1975: 'I made up my mind I would help if he needed, if he asked; he didn't ask, he fought it to the end. And I would have helped him, and I would just about now be getting out of jail for it. I would have done it. He died screaming.'

Another woman describes her ninety-six-year-old aunt's disastrous condition. 'She had a massive stroke when she was ninety-three, is bedridden completely, she knows nothing and all I want is the feeding tube to be removed from her, and they will not do it. The nursing home has told me to get her out of there if I want this done. The doctor has threatened me that he will get off the case and they just will not, and the poor thing is just suffering, just terribly.'

This theme is picked up by another woman: 'The best advice that I got, and it seems the best advice that doctors feel they can give, is *Do not put a terminal patient in the hospital*, because you lose all control over them. You have no choice in the matter then. Once they're put on survival you can't take them off.' This is a questionable assertion, given the Karen Ann Quinlan and Nancy Cruzan cases, but the struggles involved may well seem impossible. And in fact, too, the nursing home proposed an option to the niece of the ninety-six-year-old stroke patient: take her out of the institution. The niece does not see it as an option, because it is very hard to do emotionally, but she could take her aunt home under hospice care, or have her discharged to a hospice in some communities. There the feeding tube could be removed and her aunt made comfortable while dying. But few families have the strength to do this when, as in this case, the doctor looking after the patient is strongly opposed.

A man in his fifties speaks forcefully of his Native American roots:

I come from an Indian background, and even back in those days, even then, they knew what to do and when it was time to go. The point is when they knew it was time to go, no one interfered with them. You left camp, everyone knew where you were going, or what area or spot you had picked ahead of time. And no one interfered. Call it what you want, but no one interfered. You decided. You knew when it was time to go. You might sit there for several days before you finally go, but no one touched that spot and no one interfered. Because *you* decided that it was time to go. I think man is the only animal that finally outsmarted Mother Nature. And in outsmarting Mother Nature I think he kind of outsmarted himself.

Another man says matter of factly, 'When my quality of life is no longer happy to me, I'm gonna leave.' But as another woman points out, 'The trouble is it has to be legalized, because you can be ready to go and you've got the medicine right there, but you can't do it.' The man mistakenly thinks she is talking about will. 'You can't,' she goes on, 'I mean if you are not physically able to reach over there and get the medication and take it, and no one can help you.' 'I want to go before that,' the man says, but, as the woman again sees, it's not that simple. 'That makes people feel they'll do it before it's really necessary, because they're afraid tomorrow . . . I mean you look at me here today – tomorrow I may be lying there comatose. You know, every one of us could, and it's too late then. Should I do it today, instead of cuttin' the grass?'

Her witty line penetrates to the heart of the problem. The decision to die is not one we want to take lightly, but the longer we put it off the greater the chance that we will be physically or mentally incapable of acting just at the moment when we would most want to act. Then we have stumbled into Hamlet's 'calamity of too long life'. People want to die with dignity, and they are afraid that they will not be allowed to do so. One white-haired lady spoke forcefully: 'By this age I would rather be a dog. When their time comes, they just get a hypo. In minutes – in practically seconds – you're asleep, and it's finished! What is the big deal about human beings being dragged on and on with excruciating pain? It's ridiculous!'

On the table in the room are copies of Derek Humphry's best-selling book, *Final Exit*, which gives both practical advice about and ethical justification for suicide, including assisted suicide, in the setting of painful or humiliating terminal illness. Legislative initiatives have been made in California, Washington State and elsewhere to decriminalize assisted suicide and even euthanasia. Michigan, which has no law against assisted suicide, has recently become something of a haven for a non-clinical physician, Doctor Jack Kevorkian – a pathologist – who has invented a suicide machine. With it, he has aided in the suicide of at least four women with degenerative terminal illnesses. In the first of these cases a grand jury was convened, but it refused to indict him on any charges whatever. Although he has flaunted his disregard for court orders, assisting in several other suicides, it is still not clear that he will be punished. The state is presently appealing the decision but in 1992 a lower court in Michigan dismissed murder charges against Kevorkian in two more of the deaths.

Similar exoneration closed the case of Doctor Timothy Quill in New York State, after his admission – in a leading medical journal, followed by his self-identification some months later – that he had acceded to the request of 'Debbie', a young terminal patient in pain, by placing a lethal overdose of barbiturates near her bed. It was in that same journal that twelve prominent US physicians, representing different specialties and regions of the country, admitted that practices such as Doctor Quill's are in fact widespread, and that most of them did not disapprove. Poll after poll among ordinary citizens – in Britain and other countries, as well as the US – shows a steadily growing public approval of them as well.

But Carlos Gomez's study in the Netherlands raises questions about the practices, questions that come into the realm of practical ethics. Daniel Callahan, too, fears the release of an army of doctors who, feeling that they have a licence to kill, may privately play god. And this is not a role they are likely to relish. For all the assurance of some patients that they have a right to demand a lethal injection from the doctor, doctors too have rights. And they may well resist such formidable demands on their consciences, having spent their working lives struggling to stave off death. We may not have the right to ask doctors to bring death about. But the question of whether suicide, including assisted suicide, is ethical is separable from the question of whether doctors should be involved in such acts. And the debate on these issues will doubtless continue.

Callahan's solution of ceasing major intervention after a universal cut-off age is unlikely to be adopted, because the differences among the elderly of a given age are simply too large. If it is a great ethical burden to discriminate among the elderly to determine who, on purely biological grounds, is the best candidate for say, heroic resuscitation measures, it is at least an equally great ethical burden to condemn the elderly across the board to be deprived of resuscitation. Indeed, as Christine Cassel has said, it might in effect leave us morally crippled. We might find ourselves resembling those German intellectuals, a jurist and a psychiatrist, who wrote in 1920 of 'lives devoid of value' – a prelude to some of the most devastating immoralities of our destructive and insensitive century.

Yet eventually there is always a time for dying. The people of North India come to the holy city of Benares on the Ganges when they believe the time has come for them to die. Benares, they believe, is the home of Lord Shiva, the high god who presides over happiness. Although they will often avail themselves of what the hospital there has to offer – including high-powered Western medicine not available at all twenty years ago – they do not come for that, but for 'a good death'. According to Hindu belief, if you die in Benares near the banks of the Ganges, you die in a state of grace – and your soul is released from the reincarnation cycle of life and death. You no longer have to be born and die, only to be born again, as all those who die in less exalted states do, but you pass on to heaven. This is in effect synonymous with 'a good death', and it is certainly not one in which the body is poked full of needles and tubes surrounded by busy strangers. Indeed, such a death may be seen as a torture of the body. A patient in hospital whose life can no longer be prolonged by the efforts of doctors and nurses is discharged to the care of the family.

Grown children pay back their 'parental debt' by making a good death possible for their mothers and fathers. One family has already attended to the dying of their father in Benares; their mother, Mata Shukla, is now dying here. She is conscious and able to speak a little, but the doctors have said that she will not live long. They have discharged her from the hospital to a special place for the dying, where her family surrounds her, and chants to Krishna are being sung in the next room. Her daughter-in-law bathes her, while the dying woman awaits the imminent arrival of her eldest son. Another relative brings her sugar dissolved in water, and another gently banters with her about food. She complains a little of pain in her shoulders, and suggests at one point, perhaps jokingly, that she might go for a ride in a cart 'to look around'. No one is thinking about postponing this death, and yet no one is in the slightest hurry. Their job is to wait and watch, to make her feel comfortable, and to weave a kind of spiritual burial cloth out of love, filial obligation and caring.

After her death – twelve days after arriving in Benares – she is dressed in an actual burial cloth, a beautiful one draped with garlands, and borne through the streets of Benares on a platform carried on the shoulders of her relatives. While musicians play and her loved ones cast rice – the symbol of life – over her body, the dense crowd parts before the procession down to the Ganges. Here, as dusk falls, the cremation fires are lit. Her ashes are scattered over the holy river. Her heirs can now return to their village to go on with their earthly lives knowing that they have done the right thing.

Whatever our own version of 'a good death' – and it is very probably different from a good death in Benares – it is not likely to be one where the dying person is being almost assaulted in a hospital by well-meaning strangers brandishing medical technology – weapons against disease that may well have once been appropriate but may no longer be so. And if we hope to have a good death, in whatever culture we live in, we will somehow need to know when to put an end to the assault.

CHAPTER 8

PANDEMIC

Today AIDS is a household word, and one that inspires almost universal fear. Everyone, it seems, knows that it is incurable and fatal, that average men and women can avoid it by abstaining from sex, and can reduce their chances of getting it by changing sex partners as little as possible and by using condoms. Even most intravenous drug users know that they are at high risk of contracting it by sharing needles.

Yet rates of this devastating disease are rising rapidly in almost all countries and exponentially in the world as a whole. As of 1992 in the United States, where the disease was first identified in 1981, there have been 250 000 cases and 130 000 deaths, and it is projected that there will be one million cases by the turn of the millennium – all of which, barring a 'miracle cure', will end in death by the year 2010. By that date, barring a vaccine, there may be millions of cases more. At least one in four babies – perhaps as many as one in two – born to infected mothers are themselves infected, and none of these children will live to grow up.

In the world as a whole, according to 1992 World Health Organization estimates, there are about twelve million people infected – most not yet sick – including a million children; by the year 2000 there will be forty million. These are conservative estimates; some recent private projections by scientists – who think that WHO has political reasons to underestimate the problem – have been up to three times higher. But even taking the lower figure of forty million, if, as seems quite possible, this number roughly quadruples again in each of

the first two decades of the twenty-first century, then around one in ten people in the world will be infected.

Moreover, ninety per cent of current cases worldwide, according to WHO, were acquired by heterosexual transmission, a picture that belies the ideas that AIDS is largely restricted to male homosexuals and drug addicts. According to US Surgeon General Antonia Novello, there are only an eighth as many American women as men who are infected – which indicates a low level of heterosexual transmission – but among teenagers, more than a third of those infected are girls. This latter pattern is more similar to that found in Central and East Africa, where *no* groups are protected from the virus, except perhaps those who are no longer sexually active. Unborn children are a prime risk group in Africa.

According to recent studies of teenagers entering US Job Corps programmes, the ratio of infected girls to infected boys is about equal. This incidence is because more than half of all teenagers become sexually active before finishing high school and most of them do not use condoms. So even if parents do not pass on AIDS to their children at birth, the chances of children contracting the disease in adolescence are increasing steadily, and if they do, they will almost certainly be dead before they are thirty.

In Britain, according to epidemiologist Anne M. Johnson, writing in the *British Medical Journal* in May 1992, there is also a heterosexual epidemic looming on the horizon. The British epidemic is heavily influenced by travel to Commonwealth countries where the spread of AIDS has been predominantly heterosexual for a decade. In England, Wales and Northern Ireland, between 1986 and 1991, 'the proportion of cases of AIDS attributable to heterosexual transmission increased from two per cent to fourteen per cent and of diagnosed HIV infections, from four per cent to twenty-three per cent'. Of those British HIV infections acquired heterosexually, only seventeen per cent came through sex with someone in a high risk category, for example, an intravenous drug user or a bisexual man. The remaining eighty-three per cent were infected by what is called secondary or 'second generation' heterosexual transmission, that is, they got it heterosexually from someone who also got it heterosexually. Although the numbers are still very small, with only 1620 people infected in this way by the end of 1991, they are rapidly on the rise.

The notion of who is at risk in the UK is constantly evolving. In the early 1980s the only group considered at risk were gay men who had had partners in the US. Today promiscuous heterosexuals are also seen as at risk. As Johnson concludes, 'Prospective sexual partners do

not come with a log book of their past partners and experiences ...
Perhaps the most important lesson to be learnt from the accounts of
second generation heterosexual transmission in the United Kingdom
is that many of those infected did not perceive themselves as at risk.'

Meanwhile in the US, a new epidemic has begun alongside the
AIDS epidemic: tuberculosis has been on the rise again since 1988 –
ironically, the same year that the TB unit of the Centers for Disease
Control optimistically changed its name from 'TB Control' to 'TB
Elimination'. It is far from being eliminated now. Not only are the
number of cases rapidly increasing, but many of the new cases are
resistant to all drugs known up to now to be effective in TB. These
strains evolved because of failure by some patients to complete the full
and rather long course of treatment for the older strains of TB, the
kind the drugs cured. Following the process described in an earlier
chapter, the restless tide of resistant TB microbes surged into the gaps
left by inadequate use of the old barriers.

In Britain too there has recently been a big rise in tuberculosis,
which has increased by ten per cent in the five years from 1987 to
1991, and by fifteen per cent among young women from 1987 to
1989. A research project in Liverpool by Dr Peter Davies, consultant
in respiratory diseases at Sefton Hospital, Liverpool, revealed that the
highest levels of tuberculosis were among the poorest areas of the city,
and there seems little doubt of the link between poverty and the rise
in TB.

Thus the AIDS pandemic – a term for an epidemic that persists,
eventually becoming pervasive in a large population, or for parallel
epidemics around the world – may now be complicated by an epidemic
of one of the classic killers of history, and one that worldwide still
causes more deaths than any other infectious disease. Unlike AIDS,
TB is not contracted in an obvious way: the TB microbes are borne
through the air on tiny droplets, droplets often coughed out by
sufferers. And unlike AIDS, when TB kills (as it often does if it is a
drug-resistant strain), it kills quickly. Moreover, patients infected with
AIDS may have TB, yet still test negative for it, since AIDS affects
the body's immune system and may thus prevent the typical response
in the TB test.

It is of course always possible that a cure or a vaccine for AIDS
will be found. But according to the most optimistic projections, tens
of millions more will contract the infection, and millions who now
carry the virus will develop the disease and die before either solution
comes to pass.

There are some formidable obstacles to both prevention and cure.

The AIDS virus itself is remarkably hardy and adaptable. Although it was not discovered until the 1980s, two cases have been identified as likely to have been AIDS as early as the 1950s. The virus probably lay dormant long before that, possibly for centuries. The theory is that it emerged and spread in Africa because of population movements due to civil war, urbanization and consequent changes in social behaviour; while internationally the frequency of air travel has been a major factor. By the time the human epidemic was beginning, the virus was able to exist in many slightly different forms. This indeed appears to be an important key to its success – the body's immune system is essentially outrun by the virus's changeability. Various forms of the virus are present in about equal numbers during the early stages of the disease, but as the body's immune system becomes exhausted, the forms that reproduce fastest begin to predominate and can no longer be contained. Drugs like AZT and DDI, both of which at first looked very promising, are outrun in a similar way and amount in the end to temporary delaying tactics. Many conceivable future drugs and vaccines can probably be circumvented by this remarkable virus in a similar way.

The situation is not hopeless; new tactics are being tried and an effective cure or vaccine may eventually be discovered. But the AIDS virus itself is a prime example of the 'restless tide' metaphor, and it has already dashed the hopes of many infected people who had thought they might outlive the epidemic. The virus's evolution under natural conditions prepared it to fight off many forces arrayed against it, and the forces deployed by medical science so far have apparently not afforded it any surprises. There is no magic bullet for AIDS in the offing; most scientists expect that drugs will be perfected for treatment only in the long term.

That means that the only way to save lives is to slow the spread of the virus from person to person. As columnist Charles Krauthammer has said, AIDS is the quintessential behavioural epidemic. With the exception of the unborn, and of those who contracted the virus from infected blood transfusions, almost all cases have resulted from sexual activity (especially unprotected vaginal or anal intercourse) or from needle sharing among intravenous drug users. These patterns have resulted in some religious groups concluding that AIDS is a punishment for sin – don't sin, they claim, and you won't get it. Jehovah's Witnesses are even able to include transfusion in this concept, since they are forbidden to accept this frequently life-saving intervention.

This blame-the-victim moralizing is as unhelpful as it is illogical – if AIDS is God's punishment for male homosexuals, then lesbians must be among God's chosen people, since they have lower rates of infection than heterosexuals. But translating the religious idea into public health terms, we do have to recognize – not blame, but recognize – the role of human action in this disease.

AIDS is the first epidemic in which civil rights, in particular the individual's right to medical confidentiality, have taken precedence over at least some public health considerations. Some voices have been raised in the medical and public health communities calling for more widespread testing, as well as for modifications of confidentiality when an infected individual is placing others at risk, but the issue is highly contentious, centring as it does on people's private sex lives. In Britain, it has been legally very difficult for physicians and health officials to keep records identifying infected individuals. Still, the police are keeping such records on criminals as a means of protecting their own personnel, who may have to arrest and otherwise deal with infected people – a procedure that has survived legal challenge. Many have claimed that abrogating civil liberties would in every instance worsen the situation by driving victims underground; others argue that such a risk must be weighed against other risks, and against the benefits to be gained. It is highly likely that this debate will intensify in the future, especially given the ancillary epidemic of drug-resistant TB, which is more communicable than AIDS.

Regardless of how this debate evolves, the fundamental causes of the AIDS epidemic lie in conditions that are outside the control of those who contract the virus and spread it. The situation is similar to that encountered by Rudolph Virchow and other physicians in the social medicine movement during the nineteenth century as they tried to make sense of the epidemics of that era. They were dealing with diseases that they sensed were caused by microbes – and eventually were proved to be so – but it was clear that social conditions played an essential role in spreading the diseases.

What these conditions had in common was poverty. Overcrowding, poor nutrition, ignorance and hopelessness favoured alcohol and drug abuse then as it does now. The countless humiliations of poverty in that society as in ours left sex, drinking and drugs as virtually the only escapes from the hopelessness of life in a prison with no exit. Then as now some sanctimonious people who had never had to deal with real poverty themselves insisted on blaming the victims, and so a broad religious coalition concluded that the root cause of epidemics was sin. As the century drew to a close the microbe theorists were in the ascendance and the sin theorists on the wane. But in fact both microbial spread and sin stemmed from the same roots: poverty, overcrowding, malnutrition, ignorance and despair.

Thailand, for example, like most Asian countries is overcrowded and struggling to overcome the problems of underdevelopment. Like countries, rich and poor, anywhere in the world, it has always had a sex trade. But during the war in Vietnam, when men serving in the US and allied forces in the region went to Thailand for 'R & R' – some called it 'I & I', for Intoxication and Intercourse – sex for sale became routine, and in the years since it became deeply entrenched and institutionalized. Prostitution reached down through teenagers to enlist twelve-year-olds and less. Rural poverty and desperation disgorged thousands of such children into the cities, there to be bought and sold not just night by night or trick by trick, but on a very long-term basis, as indentured 'servants' with little hope of release from the brothels holding their bonds.

By the late 1980s, with AIDS on the rise in most of the world, Bangkok was a mecca for sex tourists – Japanese, Australian and European men who flew there expressly to purchase the favours of Thailand's increasingly famous prostitutes. In 1988 there were very few cases of reported AIDS in the country, and even intravenous drug users showed only a one or two per cent rate of infection with the virus. There were many advance warnings but there were few precautions taken, and Thailand today has one of the highest HIV positive rates in the world.

Approximately 400 000 people are infected in a nation of about fifty million. The projections are that by 1996 the country will have some 90 000 full-blown cases of AIDS – and that will be just the beginning. But there are now only 100 000 hospital beds in the entire country. Buddhist monks are distributing condoms and preparing to care for thousands of AIDS patients in their monasteries. In some regions seventy per cent of the busy prostitutes are HIV positive, and they will act as a reservoir for the spread of the epidemic throughout the country, and to Japan, Australia and Europe, from which some five million men a year come to Bangkok looking for illicit sex. As one observer described the public health situation with respect to AIDS in Thailand, it is like an air raid in which the sirens have sounded but the bombs have not yet dropped.

Doctor Praphan, of the Chulalongkorn Hospital in Bangkok, saw the first case of AIDS in Thailand in an American homosexual man early in 1985. Today he sees fifty to sixty people a day in his HIV clinic. In the early years they were mostly homosexuals or bisexuals who were affected, but by the late 1980s the great majority had acquired the virus through intravenous drug use; now, Doctor Praphan estimates, about ninety per cent of the new cases stem from heterosexual intercourse. Thus in three or four years Thailand has run through a cycle that is taking over a decade in Western countries.

Since the poor are more often driven by circumstances to become sex workers, and since the poorer customers are more likely to frequent poorer prostitutes – in turn more likely to be infected – AIDS is spreading most rapidly among the poor. Yet there are recent hints of some slowing in the rate of spread of the infection. Prostitutes when interviewed show considerable understanding of how AIDS is transmitted, and they know that condoms can reduce the chance of transmission. Some claim to be asking, and getting, their clients to use protection – although since the government economizes by not giving out jelly with the condoms, intercourse becomes abrasive and painful, discouraging condom use. Still, these small positive signs are the result of what, for a poor country, has been a massive government effort at education for prevention. One Thai physician sums it up:

> We're probably the first in the world to pull in the police to help campaign against AIDS and promote condoms. We're probably the first in the world to have the biggest campaign on changing sexual culture. In terms of medicine itself we have gone through a lot, educating medical personnel and trying to change the philosophy of medicine, to move from just medicine into society; move from the virus into the human being.

As a result, many have come to think of Thailand as 'the biggest classroom on AIDS prevention in the world'.

In the north, towards the Burmese border, terraced green hills slope down and level off in vast rice paddies; men and women stand knee-deep in water, tending the plants that have kept them alive for thousands of years, while water buffalo plod by in the service of that same ancient goal. Women here have always played a key role in supporting their families, so it is easy to understand how young girls may find it difficult to resist ensuring the survival of their families by selling their bodies for what must seem to them great riches. Doctor Wat, of the region's Chiang Rai Hospital, takes prostitution for granted as he tries to think of ways to slow the spread of AIDS in his country.

A dedicated and compassionate man – he has taken in three children orphaned by AIDS – Doctor Wat pursues the general practice of medicine in this beautiful countryside where, he knows, the population goes about its daily business unaware that it is about to be ravaged by AIDS. He tries to convince young women infected with the virus to have their tubes tied, so as not to give birth to children who, even if they are lucky enough to escape the disease, will certainly be orphaned when they are less than half grown. He patiently cares for the early victims of the epidemic, who have developed the burdensome symptoms and begun the long, painful process of dying. But in keeping with his belief that 'every doctor should be involved in prevention', he spends time visiting the brothels.

These are not as dangerous in Chiang Rai as in Bangkok, and the one he visits regularly has an almost festive atmosphere. Girls – mostly in their teens – attend a kind of survival school run by Doctor Wat and his colleagues, where the girls banter and giggle about the toys they have been given to play with. These particular toys give new meaning to the phrase 'educational playthings.' They are crudely carved wooden dolls with removable barrels around them; the barrel, the girls learn, is like the clothes on one of their customers – entirely superficial – and to find out what is underneath the clothes – the real man – you pull off the barrel. Out pop a couple of stick-arms and a penis even larger and thicker than the arms. On some of the dolls, near the tip of the penis is a big red spot, vivid against the dull wood. That spot represents the disease that the well-dressed man with the fistful of money can give the girl, a disease that will cause her and her children to die.

Other 'toys' are used to teach the girls how to use condoms to try to avert this fate, and according to Doctor Wat, condom use has reached very high levels – he believes one hundred per cent – in this particular brothel. While this figure may be overly optimistic, it is likely that his programme has had an impact, and in the face of such a rapidly growing menace, even a slowing down in the rate of spread is a goal to be eagerly sought.

Unfortunately, the Thai government is beginning to discourage these dedicated physicians by greatly toning down the already successful AIDS awareness campaign. At issue is the country's tourist industry, worth about 2.5 billion pounds sterling annually. The number of tourists dropped to 5.1 million in 1991, alarming some government officials and leading to the conclusion that the AIDS awareness campaign had been *too* successful. The sex industry itself, only part of which is tourist-supported, is a billion-pound-a-year business. It is estimated that ninety per cent of Thai men participate in it at some point in their lives.

Yet given the Bangkok Metropolitan Association estimate that thirty-seven per cent of the city's prostitutes are infected, a figure that rises to seventy per cent in the north, it seems amazing that AIDS awareness would be deliberately curtailed at this time. Even in purely economic terms, it seems irrational to try to protect a three-billion-pound-a-year economic sector in ways that will ultimately threaten the entire economy of what has been until now one of the most effective of all developing countries. But it is happening, and it is only one of the baffling paradoxes with which AIDS confronts us.

Another such paradox is the fact that AIDS, in common with other human disasters from which great insights have sometimes arisen, has forced physicians and public health officials to take an approach to its prevention that has not been seen since the heyday of the social medicine movement of the nineteenth century. As Doctor Jonathan Mann, former director of the World Health Organization's AIDS prevention programmes, summarized it at the Sixth International Conference on AIDS which was held in 1990, 'AIDS is catalyzing a revolution in health care.'

> No one set out to make a revolution . . . yet, in carrying forward this work, the deficiencies of our health care and social systems worldwide have been so starkly and painfully revealed that the pre-AIDS era paradigm of health care, its philosophy and practice, has been challenged and found to be desperately inadequate and, therefore, fatally obsolete . . . The emphasis was medical and technological, involving experts and engineers, and, for certain purposes, this approach was quite effective. However, this paradigm envisioned a fundamental dichotomy between individual and social interests . . . Attention to behavioural, social and societal considerations was often rudimentary and naive . . .

He goes on to describe the enormous impact that the worldwide fight against AIDS has made on this old approach. 'The key to the new paradigm is the recognition that behaviour, both individual and collective, is the major public health challenge of the future.'

Doctor Mann also notes that AIDS has shrunk the worldwide network of medicine and health, because the epidemic itself is the product of a shrunken world. 'For example,' he points out, 'international travel has increased fifteen-fold since 1950,' reflecting 'an increasingly global linkage and interdependence. This also offers infectious agents an unparalleled opportunity for rapid pandemic spread; HIV may be the first virus to take advantage of this situation, but it is unlikely to be the last.'

This global solidarity, for better or for worse, helps bring thousands of tourists a month to Thailand, where their wealth buys sybaritic pleasures to match their wildest dreams. It also buys them AIDS. However, this international commerce in viruses is not a one-way street; on the contrary. Just as the rich countries export to the poor ones such things as cigarettes that give them epidemics of heart disease and lung cancer, and weapons that make possible wholesale slaughter of their own and neighbouring peoples, so we send them tourists who, in the mid-1980s, brought Thailand its first cases of AIDS.

These particular tourists almost certainly came from the United States and Australia. Australia, in fact, helped pioneer the AIDS pandemic, with rates in the mid-1980s that were higher than in almost any other country. Sydney, a city with all the ills of any modern metropolis – poverty, drug abuse, prostitution, violent crime – initially had a large number of AIDS cases because, like San Francisco in the US, it has a large gay population. Many of these men had become infected before 1985, just as among American gays. Yet Australia has not had a second phase of the AIDS epidemic nearly as large as that in the US.

This second phase consists of the spread of the disease among drug users through the sharing of contaminated needles, followed by its spread through heterosexual sex with non-drug-using partners – often by prostitutes who are also drug users. These are people on the margins of society, with less access to health care, money, information, psychological and social support – everything. They have generally grown up less educated, more abused and neglected, less well nourished, impoverished in every way, than other children. They care less about risk and danger because they have less to live for, and because risky pleasures take them away, at least for a moment, from the depressing conditions of their lives.

They may also not believe what they are told about the dangers. An American study in 1992 of poor black youth at risk from AIDS showed that their mistrust of establishment figures, indeed all adults, is so great that what they hear from them about the threat of AIDS is often simply discounted, especially when it conflicts with what they hear from their risk-prone, frequently ignorant peers. Even the earnest and powerful warnings of their long-standing hero 'Magic' Johnson, the great basketball player who is open about being HIV-positive, are ignored; they see even him as having sold out and become an untrustworthy part of the establishment.

So how is it that their counterparts in Australia – admittedly mainly white, but otherwise similar in background, deprivation, marginalization and risk, are not travelling the same fast road towards a high prevalence of AIDS? The answer may lie with the actions of a surprisingly small number of dedicated, courageous doctors and other health care workers who have gone into the streets and somehow made these young people believe them. One of them is Doctor Alex Wodak, who treated some of the first AIDS cases in Australia in 1982. He still finds clinical medicine – treatment, the medical care of the ill – the most satisfying work he does, yet confronted with the growing number of AIDS victims in Sydney, he concluded that he had to do more. He explains:

> It just seemed not enough to look after individual patients. There's a very great figure in public health called John Snow, who was involved in trying to control the cholera epidemic in London. He traced the epidemic down to a particular water pump in Soho. And when he worked out what was going on – worked out that the cholera was spreading from that water pump – he pulled the handle off that pump so that people couldn't use the well, and that stopped the epidemic. And he's really held up as a model by people like me, who think that it's not enough to treat the diarrhoea of people who have cholera. You've got to do something about controlling epidemics at their source.
>
> So for me it was very clear that we had to distribute clean needles and syringes.

He makes this transition from cholera to AIDS, from John Snow's water-pump handle to his own needle-exchange programme, sound easy, which is far from the truth. No one accused Snow of debasing the morals of London's poor by disabling a contaminated water pump, but Doctor Wodak was open to accusations of corrupting morals, in the same way Paul Ehrlich had been for introducing his cure for syphilis. Needle exchange, many were convinced, would only increase the number of addicts – a prediction much evidence has since con-tradicted. Doctor Wodak had first to confront the police force of Sydney and then the government of Australia. A mild-looking, soft-spoken man, he is, like most physicians, not of a mind to become a law-breaker, and he and his colleagues at the hospital went through official channel after official channel:

> Finally, I got frustrated with all this sort of committee work and writing more and more reports and documents. So I went to my colleagues in my department and I said, 'We're getting nowhere, and

everyone's afraid to break the ice, and somebody's going to have to do it without any permission. Let's do it – let's do it with our own money, let's do it on our own time. So that's what we did . . . we put a notice on the door November the thirteenth, 1986. And we started, and people came, and we handed out needles and syringes, and the press came in droves . . .

And then the next year they changed the law so that what we were doing was no longer illegal.

Asked if he thinks it the role of the doctor to break the law, he says nervously, 'No, I – I'd only do it in epidemics . . . I just figured that a doctor has a lot of privileges, and if you can't use your position in – in society . . . now and then, when it really matters, if you can't use your position to force something that has to happen, then you shouldn't really have those privileges.' He speaks too of 'a totally different form of medicine than we would have been practising a generation or two generations ago'.

We're now dealing mainly with lifestyle problems over which individuals have at least some control, and we have to maximize that control . . . We're also dealing now, more and more in Western medicine, with chronic diseases which relapse, and remitting diseases that come and go. We're not dealing with sort of flash point acute episodes where the doctor comes in on the white horse and lances the boil and everything's alright.

Over a century ago Rudolph Virchow said, 'Politics is only medicine on a grand scale.' Today Alex Wodak says, 'You can't separate medicine and politics. They are sides of the same coin.' He recognizes that politics, even if it is a form of medicine, is not a satisfying or appealing form; but he stresses the need for changes in medical training. Indeed, he seems to be calling for a new kind of doctor. What he says is not so different from what Johns Hopkins intern John Townes said after treating Isabel Humbles at the end of her long course of alcohol and drug abuse: it is not enough to be there at the end-point, in the crisis; the problem won't be solved there, it has to be solved earlier, before things get that bad. But Wodak, an experienced physician, practising in an environment more conducive to change, sounds far more hopeful.

And he is not alone. Doctor Rachael Buckley and Doctor Ingrid Van Beek practise the new kind of medicine at the Kirketon Road Centre in 'the Cross' – the King's Cross section of Sydney where male and female prostitutes and drug addicts converge with droves of middle-class suburban youth out on the town for a thrill. And not just youth: according to one HIV-positive male prostitute hanging out at 'The Wall', a centre of sex-for-sale in the city, more than half of the men who do business with him have children's car seats in their vehicles. These middle-class youths and family men have the potential to carry the AIDS epidemic throughout Australian society.

Yet so far that spread is not happening. Doctor Buckley and Doctor Van Beek, along with others staffing the Centre, are effectively standing in the way of it. They never thought when they went into medicine that this was what they would be doing. Night after night they climb aboard the AIDS Bus – which sallies forth in the late hours seven nights a week – and go to the source of the problem, like John Snow homing in on the Soho water pump. They give out 5000 clean needles and syringes a week. They stock condoms too by the thousands. They teach ignorant teenagers toying with their lives how to stay alive a few years longer – maybe long enough for them to turn to lifestyles less likely to destroy them. They teach them how to clean needles with bleach so as to kill the AIDS virus, and how to persuade customers to use condoms. They try to convince already infected young women not to become pregnant and pass the disease on to an unborn child.

What they don't do is judge, having learned that that is no way to slow an epidemic. Their strategy is called harm reduction or harm minimization. The assumption is that these young people will keep on doing harmful things, that they cannot be prohibited from doing them, and that in many cases they cannot be cured of doing them; all a doctor or health worker can hope to do is reduce the harm they will do themselves by engaging in such behaviour. The work may not be as satisfying, or as easy, as lancing boils, but where AIDS is concerned it saves a lot more lives. They don't have the gratification of effecting a simple cure, but they can watch the number of AIDS cases in Australia begin to level off, while the number in the United States and Britain continues to rise and rise again.

Doctor van Beek even tries to convince patients who inject cocaine to switch to heroin. It seems an odd role for a doctor. But an intravenous heroin user may need to inject only once or twice a day, while an intravenous cocaine user may need to inject twenty times. If she persuades her patient to switch, she reduces that person's risk of contracting AIDS from a dirty needle by ninety or ninety-five per cent; harm reduction, indeed.

In Perth, the Western Australian Health Department is actually paying a salary to prostitutes who carry the AIDS virus, on condition that they stop selling sex. And the Australian national government distributes a highly explicit, even obscene comic called *Streetwize*, which assumes that young people are mainlining drugs and having all kinds and combinations of licit and illicit sex. Despite being a government publication, *Streetwize* speaks the language of risk-prone youth, improper and often unpleasant though it may be to others. Rather than preaching, it gives them role models who are 'cool' and 'down and dirty' but who use bleach and condoms because they intend to stay alive, and it portrays those who don't as uncool numskulls. A prison version of the comic, *Gaolwize*, directs similar information and persuasion at inmates, many of whom are known to engage in homosexual sex and inject drugs while in prison.

All these efforts at education are carried out at Australian government expense. They could not conceivably be done in the United States or, probably, Britain, although there are some needle-exchange programmes in Britain, and some family planning clinics – now being reduced in number by the government – give out condoms to young people. This seems especially peculiar given the evidence that harm minimization works well in the UK. Studies of HIV infection among drug users in Edinburgh during the mid-1980s showed large increases, apparently due to legal discouragement of needle-exchange programmes in Scotland. But in comparable cities in Wales, Northern Ireland and England – Liverpool, for example – where needle exchange had been instituted, no such increase took place during the same period.

But to reward prostitutes by paying them a salary to avoid sex, to teach law-breaking addicts how to do injections safely, to admit openly that there is sex and drugs in prisons – any of this would be seen as condoning crime and immorality; better to pretend and preach. Accordingly, American and British prostitutes will continue to ply their trade, spreading the virus far and wide. In the US needle-sharing without precautions will go on apace – Louis Sullivan, the US Secretary of Health and Human Services, in 1992 killed another attempt to fund clean-needle programmes – and the second phase of the epidemic will accelerate. And American prisons will discharge tens of thousands of AIDS-infected people into the community over the next few years.

This is what might be called the Ostrich Strategy, which we carry forward while the Australian government practises harm reduction. We will have hundreds of thousands of unnecessary cases of AIDS – but the gratification of knowing that we held firm to our high moral standards.

Dade County, where Miami is, has perhaps the highest rate of HIV infection in the United States. It is fifty per cent black, twenty per cent Hispanic, and thirty per cent 'Anglo' – which really means 'other'. Doctor Joe Greer, a Cuban-American who is the Director of the Camillus Health Concern for the Homeless, serves a particular sub-group of the Dade County poor – those who have nothing to call home except a space on a street, under a bridge, on a bench or in an alleyway. In the late 1980s these people had no health – or other – services of any kind. But by the early 1990s, thanks to Doctor Greer and a few other people generous with their time, skill, medical equipment, furniture and hard cash, the Dade County homeless had some thread-bare but badly needed clinics devoted exclusively to them.

Greer himself goes prowling under the bridges and in the alleyways, in his white coat and with his stethoscope. He is a large, charismatic man, whom everyone seems to know, and he certainly knows them; they greet him unthreateningly, as a valued friend. Not only is he making house calls, he is making house calls to people who have no house. Doctor Greer has paying patients – the well-insured – in his part-time practice; in the remainder of his working time he tends to homeless people for free.

Among other serious diseases, many of these people are going to get AIDS: more than twelve per cent of the adults were HIV positive in 1990. Yet the homeless no longer fit the old generalizations about them as male 'bums' or 'hobos' who have hit the skids. A surprising number are educated, some are even college graduates. Of the esti-mated 8000 homeless people in Miami alone, approximately a third are women, and contrary to the 'bag lady' stereotype, their average age is twenty-three. Many are pregnant or caring for dependent children; roughly half of those children are under five years old, and many already have established chronic illnesses. The population of homeless in the US may be increasing by as much as twenty-five per cent a year. At that rate of compounded interest, given the high rate of AIDS infection, in no time there will be a vast harvest of death.

And it will be non-discriminating. As Doctor Greer says of his AIDS research, 'We showed no difference statistically for HIV infec-tion in the homeless, regardless of race, ethnicity, risk groups (intravenous drug abuse, prostitutes and homosexuals), or lack of risk groups. Poverty was the only common denominator.'

So what does that tell you? That this disease is the same here as it is in Haiti and other regions of the world, in third world countries. So in the United States of America we have our own little third world country. Yet we're not willing to do anything about it. We're not willing to do the prevention.

AIDS is the easiest disease to visualize spreading throughout society from a reservoir among the homeless. But there are many other diseases rampant among them. Hepatitis (transmitted in ways similar to AIDS) and other sexually transmitted diseases, as well as the new forms of tuberculosis, are highly correlated with AIDS in this population.

And the homeless nationally have three times as much high blood pressure, twice as many gastrointestinal disorders, five times as many neurological disorders and ten times as much peripheral vascular disease – for example, gangrene and varicose veins, partly stemming from abnormal sleeping postures. 'In effect,' Greer says in conclusion, 'a third world country of disease is superimposed over first world country diseases. What we don't pay for today, we'll pay for tomorrow, not only economically but in the future of this country.'

Like his Australian counterparts Alex Wodak and Ingrid Van Beek, Doctor Greer is not concerned with apportioning blame or moralizing about other people's behaviour. He cares about harm reduction. And like them, he does not work alone. Bessie Garrett, for example, is an intensive care nurse who also spends a lot of time on the street, and has a remarkable knowledge about the homeless people she finds there. For instance, many people think that women are a better target for education about condoms than men, but Bessie Garrett has discovered that if she gives condoms out to women, for them to get men to use, the man may see this as a sign of the woman's infidelity and beat her up. So she usually talks to men, rather than women, about safe sex.

Dade County needs dozens of professionals like Doctor Greer and Bessie Garrett, but Americans are generally not willing to pay for them to do what they do. While it is inspiring to see individuals like these who have the courage and dedication to go against the system and give of themselves in ways that few others are prepared to emulate, what is needed is a systematic approach to training and rewarding such people. What is needed is a response from society, a willingness to make sacrifices to help these people to keep on doing their work, and, even more important, some attention to the root causes of illness, the conditions favouring it, in the culture of poverty and despair.

Doctor Greer is a plain-spoken man who uses a grim analogy to bring out the illogicality of how Americans approach these problems:

What you're seeing here in essence is the end of the river. And what I mean by that is that you can imagine a river, and a health care provider at the edge of the river, and a body floats by. He resuscitates that body, because that's what he's trained to do. Ten more float by, he becomes tired. A thousand float by, society builds a clinic. Ten thousand, we build a hospital, one million, a giant public hospital. But somewhere along the line working at the end of the river, you start to ask: why is the bridge broken? Why are people falling off? Why do they keep floating down? Why are we putting all our efforts at the end of the river, instead of repairing it upstream?

We're trained to work at the end of the river. That's what I'm trained to do. But sometimes, the rush of the water, the people, the increasing numbers, become so overwhelming that you wonder why society doesn't turn around and deal with the real core of the problem.

A number of recent analyses, including some that have survived vigorous criticism without losing their force, have shown that during the 1980s the richest few per cent of people in the United States became substantially richer, while the poor became poorer and those in the middle essentially stagnated. Unemployment worsened dramatically, directly affecting the middle class, forcing many in this group to join the poor. Every serious study of the homeless in America has shown them greatly increasing in number during the past dozen years. Similar trends are true of the UK.

The disparity between black and white, different from and super-imposed on the one between rich and poor, has remained very great during these years according to most major measures, notably excepting the number of black actors on American television. Infant mortality, maternal mortality, rates of death from all major diseases, victimization by violence, joblessness, poverty, homelessness, school segregation – all show a continuing pattern of inequality and discrimination, summarized in the title of a recent book by distinguished sociologist Andrew Hacker: *Two Nations: Black and White, Separate, Hostile, Unequal.*

But race is not the only, or even perhaps the central problem dividing Americans. At the beginning of the 1980s a swing in public opinion, which amounted to change in philosophy, made selfishness not merely acceptable but actually admirable. It was justified in terms of the 'trickle-down' concept in economics: for the rich to get richer was supposedly good for everyone, since their greed would serve as the engine of economic growth, which, when fired up, would power the whole country, benefiting the middle class and eventually the poor. George Bush in 1980 called this 'voodoo economics', and an evil spell it turned out to be. But Mr Bush has practised and defended it himself since 1988, soothing his nation with cynical bromides about 'a kinder, gentler America'. Rarely have such assurances been more at variance with reality.

The Thatcher years in Britain saw the adoption of a similar 'trickle down' economic concept and an ethos that lauded materialism and the amassing of individual wealth at the expense of the less fortunate. Britain followed the States in a national philosophy that in effect condoned an almost complete absence of compassion.

Among the consequences in the States is the fact that in an era when every other Western industrialized nation has accepted the need to provide a minimal level of universal health care, the US has not only allowed the poor to languish in their squalor, but has forced millions more newly poor people to share that squalor with them. In an era in which most of the Communist world has recognized the superority of capitalism, the United States has failed to recognize that capitalism without compassion is a system that must ultimately sicken those who benefit from it, filling them with hesitancy and shame. And hesitancy and shame, of course, prove no sort of recipe for success.

Despite the attention we give it, the drama that surrounds our discussions of it and the unquestioned cloud it forms on the horizon, AIDS is not the most important preventable threat to health in either the developed or the underdeveloped world today. More than seventy per cent of premature deaths in the United States are attributable to three causes: smoking, inadequately treated high blood pressure and poor eating habits. Another ten per cent or so are attributable to injuries, including violence. Looking at deaths before age sixty-five, injuries loom much larger, accounting for more than forty per cent, with a major contribution from injuries caused by alcohol abuse; smoking still accounts for eighteen per cent of the deaths.

Lung cancer alone, an almost completely preventable behavioural epidemic encouraged by social, economic, political and cultural forces, will cause more than 150 000 deaths in the US in 1992 – more than the total number of AIDS deaths from 1981 to the present. This epidemic, like AIDS, affects the poor much more than it does the well-to-do; and it is only one of the major deadly diseases caused by smoking.

In general, the amount of money the US spends on AIDS research is not uncontroversial. As Doctor Robert Wachter of the University of California at San Francisco wrote in the *New England Journal of Medicine* in January 1992, 'Federal spending for AIDS was $1.6 billion in 1990, a year after 40 000 Americans died of the disease. During the same year, federal spending for cancer, a disease that killed 500 000 in 1989, was $1.5 billion, and spending for heart disease, which killed 750 000, was less than $1 billion ... in fact overall spending for health care research remained essentially fixed; it was self-evident that money spent on AIDS was money not spent on something else.' That money – or, preferably, other money – could be spent fighting cancer and heart disease through prevention programmes, which are presently lacking due to inadequate funds.

Other gaps in preventive medicine leading to needless illness and death include inadequate prenatal care, inadequate childhood immunization, inadequate mental health services, inadequate drug rehabilitation services, inadequate health education and inadequate health screening. Without exception, each of these causes of loss of life affects the poor much more than the better off; the poor have higher mortality rates in virtually every comparison. These differences are due to the same disparities in health care, knowledge and opportunity that led to large differences in mortality and illness from quite other diseases in past centuries. Then, as now, specific diseases are the mediators of the generic process: the devastating effect of poverty on health. This effect, these disparities, have been known since ancient times. We like to think that we have conquered them, put them behind us, but we certainly have not.

In the underdeveloped world, too, AIDS is not at the moment the most important killer. Tuberculosis, for instance – not the new, AIDS-related kind, but the old standby-killer – takes far more lives throughout the world than AIDS will for years to come. Malaria, with its spiking fevers and swollen bellies, strikes at least a hundred million new people a year, millions of whom die untreated or with strains resistant to the treatments we have. Tens of millions more are gravely debilitated, robbed of the vitality that makes life and work worthwhile.

Schistosomiasis, caused by a snail-borne parasite absorbed through the feet in countless bodies of water, is likewise a hopeless obstacle to vigorous life. Two hundred million people are affected worldwide by this chronic, essentially downhill disease in which bleeding occurs in internal organs ranging from the liver to the bladder, the victim loses weight, and – as in AIDS – resistance to many other diseases is lowered. Like with tuberculosis, there are drugs that help, but the course of treatment is so long that completion by the illiterate poor is very unlikely, assuming that they have access to such treatment.

About half a million women also die needlessly each year worldwide in connection with pregnancy and childbirth, most from childbed fever. This alone is still more than the number of people who will die in 1992 from AIDS worldwide, and it has occurred without stirring much excitement, year in and year out since long before the AIDS problem started.

The list of other major diseases far exceeding AIDS in their impact on the underdeveloped world could be continued at length, but it is worth mentioning three other points. First, the West is actively involved in spreading tobacco addiction to the developing world – much more rapidly and with more devastating effect than we did AIDS. In the forseeable future many more deaths will occur in Colombia from American tobacco than will occur in America from Colombian cocaine. There are 350 000 tobacco-related deaths each year in the US and 500 000 in Europe; now we are spreading this plague to developing countries. Tobacco companies, increasingly hampered by American and European health laws, are shifting their focus to a vast and vulnerable populace in the third world, where health education programmes are too impoverished to counterbalance the companies' cigarette advertising.

In Bangkok, where tobacco may ultimately do even more damage than AIDS, one advertisement reads 'Winston, Style of the USA'. American government intervention is highly unlikely given the trade deficit. As Los Angeles Congressional Representative Mel Levine has said, 'Asian lungs [are] more expendable than American lungs.' In China, women are viewing smoking as a sign of liberation, just as their European and American counterparts did in the post-war era, with continuing tragic consequences. Like AIDS, the behavioural epidemic of tobacco-caused diseases is still in an early stage in most of the developing world; unlike AIDS, nothing much is being done to slow it down.

Second, starvation – the full-blown clinical syndrome of malnutrition – affects five hundred million people a year at a minimum; some estimates range much higher. This, like AIDS, is not a pleasant way to die, and it too reduces resistance to many other diseases. To say that when countries produce more people than they can feed, many of them must starve conveniently glosses over the fact that the absence of family planning is also a public health problem – one that has been exacerbated during the past decade by ignorant Western, especially American, politicians and institutions, aided by the Catholic Church. The virtual absence of discussion of this subject at the much-vaunted Earth Summit of 1992 rendered that event almost useless, dwarfing the other criticisms levelled against it.

Third, we have virtually abandoned the world's children, leaving many to die of diseases that are easy to prevent with a small expenditure of funds. Worldwide, about fifteen million children die each year, and many millions more only survive the onslaught of illness with permanent impairment and pain. More than ten million of these fifteen million deaths are preventable with readily available measures. Diarrhoea treated with inexpensive oral rehydration salts – which an illiterate mother can easily learn to supply – would not, as it now does, lead to millions of children dying each year by simply drying up. Bacterial pneumonia and other respiratory infections, easily treatable with everyday antibiotics, would not steal the breath of life from millions more. And whooping cough, measles and tetanus – all vaccine-preventable and almost abolished from Western countries – would not ravage and kill still millions more.

Roughly 150 million – forty per cent – of the underdeveloped world's children are in the process of starving, but some other things they need are much cheaper than food. A quarter of a million children a year go blind from Vitamin A deficiency; a capsule worth a penny, given twice a year, would leave those children their sight. Untold millions suffer brain damage from iodine deficiency; for a few pence worth of iodized salt, each of them could keep the great mental and emotional powers nature has set in store for almost every human child.

So why does AIDS get so much intense attention when all these other scourges that we lack the will to wipe away remain, mocking our claims to call ourselves humane? Simply, it is because AIDS can get to *us*. It is not compassion, but fear, that has focused our attention. Annie Crowe, a non-physician who works the streets of Sydney night after night saving the lives of youngsters who don't even care to be saved, puts it very plainly:

> In the years from 1977 to the early 1980s there were no real supports for the street level at all ... I mean, you're talking about young people who are living on these streets with virtually no social supports at all, no family, no school ... no nothing, no GP, no one at all ... We had kids who were overdosing, who were suiciding, who had the most incredible range of medical problems you've ever seen, from infected tattoos through to throat infections, lung infections that turned into pneumonia before our very eyes ...
>
> Prior to AIDS I don't think anybody cared at all about street people or junkies or gays, or young street kids ... But then AIDS came and all of a sudden because of AIDS everybody got scared. Suddenly AIDS was the big virus with the street people and the money came pouring in.

Annie goes on to put these observations in an even darker light:

> Nothing, nothing in the world is worth AIDS, nothing. But the truth is that the resources that we've been able to put on these streets would not be here but for AIDS ...
>
> I mean everybody hopes and prays for a cure for AIDS. But in one sense a cure might bring our death knell here. I mean it may be that the resources do dry up if a cure was found for AIDS tomorrow ...

It is a sad irony that a person who dedicates her life, at considerable risk and with minuscule reward, to helping those whom no one else cares about – including saving them from AIDS – fears a cure for this horrible scourge because she knows that it is not the most important threat to them. And she knows too that without AIDS no one would 'give a stuff' about them, and she would be back watching them languish and die with no resources to help them, just as she was in 1980.

Although he is much less cynical than Annie Crowe, Doctor Jonathan Mann, former director of the World Health Organization's AIDS programme, has clearly made a similar reckoning. In the US as well as worldwide, spending for AIDS has for years now been far out of proportion to the share of illness and death attributable to the disease. Strong arguments can be made based on projected mortality a decade from now; but even those projections do not justify the relative neglect of other causes of premature death – many of which, even in the worst AIDS scenario, will still be more important and more damaging than AIDS after the year 2000. Yet WHO's budget for AIDS is at least double that for the next largest programme in the organization, the Tropical Disease Research Programme, which subsumes not one but a number of intrinsically more important diseases.

Mann, like Annie Crowe, is not naive. He knows that the main reason developed countries are willing to spend so much on AIDS is that they are terrified of it. And he also knows that for decades before AIDS the developed countries basically cared little about disease and death in the developing world. So although he is much more diplomatic than Crowe, he thinks something similar on a worldwide scale to what she thinks in relation to downtown Sydney. The terror of AIDS has awakened well-to-do people from their comfortable slumber and induced them to pull a few more coins – for that is all in fact it is – from their fashionable pockets, to toss at the world's continuing crisis of health. Mann and others like him are using the money to set up structures for AIDS control and prevention like the one that is working at least for now in Thailand. But they are putting these structures in places that have never had any sort of health care before, and organizing them in a new network that covers the world; and they believe that they will permanently change the process of disease control, so that long after the AIDS problem is solved the new structures will go on preventing other dreaded diseases, different needless deaths.

Let us hope that they are right. One would hope, too, that in the process we are stirred to act not only by fear for our own safety but also by the spectre of millions of painful early deaths that annually dwarf the human impact of AIDS. So far we have been incapable of responding to this challenge. But if that is the way it is, then at least let us help others out of self-interest if we cannot bring ourselves to help them out of compassion.

A NEW KIND

of DOCTOR

No doubt it is bad form for an American observer to say much about the fate of medicine and health care in Britain or other countries. But this book has ranged from Kyoto to Cleveland, from East Berlin to Sydney, from a slum in Baltimore to a brothel in Thailand, from a living room in Sun City, Arizona, to a lakeside in Italy, from Bremen to Galway, and elsewhere besides. The differences have been fascinating, and have often shed a particular light that may help us approach the future, but the common ground we are moving across is quite broad and solid.

Health care costs are rising alarmingly in America – but they are doing the same, from a lower baseline, in Britain and everywhere else. Doctors typically lie to patients in Japan – but in Western countries and elsewhere the tradition was until recently the same, and doctors continue everywhere to play their cards very close to their chests. Britain has had more experience than the US in dealing with an ageing population, but the plight of the acutely ill, elderly person probably does not tear at the social fabric any less in London than in Washington. Regardless of national boundaries, AIDS creeps from lover to lover, with or without a disapproving outsider's moral or medical gaze, and enmeshes the world in a shrinking web of con- taminated human need. Poverty, English or American, pushes victims over its jagged cliffs to float down our polluted metaphorical river, past bewildered bystanders only doing 'the right thing'. Increasingly, almost everywhere, doctors stand far downstream, less and less prepared to think and act in a timely way to stem that tragic flow of human detritus at or near its source. And the lure of the bright flashing lights and ever-more-accurate numbers on the next new piece of technology will be as compelling to young, well-trained physicians whether they hail from Miami or Riyadh, Bangkok or Siena, Sydney or Newcastle-upon-Tyne.

Consequently many countries are in danger of following America in making continually greater mess of most things medical. Young British doctors too want to play with expensive technical toys and gain the prestige that rubs off top consultants in famous teaching hospitals – not to be shared by mere GPs slogging away in their far-flung surgeries. And, of course, there are the voices calling for privatization. Unfortunately there are ominous trends away from the great tradition of national health. Beds in private hospitals and nursing homes have proliferated in England and Wales, doubling from 25 300 in 1971 to 51 000 in 1985. Available beds in NHS hospitals fell from 526 000 to 421 000 during the same period. At the level of the individual doctor, NHS economizing produces relentless pressure to process a too-large panel of patients in surgeries where five-minute visits are the norm. Even young doctors who are not dazzled by technology are becoming uncomfortable with this rushed sort of medicine; increasingly, they are succumbing to the temptation to enter private or partly private medicine, where they can not so much make more money as practise in a way that makes them feel more professional – more like doctors. Ultimately this trend could destroy the NHS.

But at the moment the mess is so much smaller in Britain than in the US that it seems stretching the point to dwell on the similarities, except as a warning. The present differences may be more telling. For example, about half the doctors in Britain remain general practitioners. In America for about the last twenty years, medical educators have tried everything they could think of to increase the number of graduating medical students who elect to stay in primary care specialties – general medicine, general paediatrics and family medicine – the latter being the rough equivalent of general practice. (It says much about the difference between Britain and the US that in America family medicine is a 'specialty' – and one not chosen very often.) Yet despite this effort, the trend in America towards specialization and sub-specialization and away from every form of primary care has continued unabated. This alone puts British medicine at an enormous advantage.

Yet Britain is in danger of losing this advantage to the universal lure of specialization and technology. In Britain as elsewhere income differences amongst different types of doctors are part of this pressure –

but only a part. After all, the young Boston doctor studying in Vienna in 1866 had felt, more than a century ago, a need to specialize, because it already seemed to him that there was too much to learn to remain a generalist. Recently I talked with a young American doctor who co-directs a very busy walk-in clinic in a big inner city hospital; she was one of the smartest students in my medical school class, but she feels she can never be really sure of herself because she has not specialized, has not focused on one subject, one set of skills. She also said that when seriously ill, as she has at times been, she wants to be cared for by an unquestioned expert, someone who has seen hundreds or thousands of very similar cases, done the required procedure hundreds or thousands of times.

This was by way of questioning the British system with its working army of general practitioners. My response was that the British plainly recognize the value of specialization; that is why half the doctors in the UK are specialists, and why an assiduously nurtured British medical science is about as good as medical science gets. It isn't a matter of devaluing specialists; it's a matter of balance – and Britain is a lot closer to the right balance than the US is.

Equally important, general practitioners are specialists too. The skills they have practised thousands of times in their surgeries are: to distinguish rapidly between life-threatening and merely frightening situations; take prompt measures to save the lives of people who have had a heart attack or taken a drug overdose, or of children with severe bleeding or epiglottitis – an inflammation that stops breathing; to sew minor lacerations in injured children without traumatizing them psychologically; to persuade patients with simple catarrh that they don't need antibiotics; to persuade busy mothers that their children need immunizations on schedule; to talk cigarettes out of the lives and lungs of a small but significant minority of patients, and, not least, to exercise day after day an increasingly learned judgement about whether to refer some patients on to more specialized doctors and keep others under a simpler regime of care. Such judgements are emphatically *not* about merely saving money for the NHS and the realm; they are also to save patients the time, trouble, discomfort, boredom, pain, side-effects and physician-induced illness that often result from the most sophisticated and specialized medical care – care that ideally should never be invoked unless it is really needed.

If the British system is no longer the envy of the world – if even those in the US who favour radical reform do not advertise the successes of the British system – it is not because it is the wrong type of organization for national health, but because only six per cent of the country's Gross Domestic Product is spent on it. The proportion of GDP spent in the US is more than double that. (Other industrial nations lie between the two in this measure: for example, Canada, France and Germany, nine per cent; Israel, eight per cent; Japan, seven per cent.) Although much of the difference is due to enormous administrative inefficiency in the US – plus substantial health care fraud, unnecessary medical and surgical procedures, cash-register physicians and runaway malpractice litigation – much of it is also due to the fact that America does more *needed* procedures, especially those based on specialization and new technology, than Britain, and does them in a more timely way.

Doctor Julian Tudor Hart, a leading figure in the Royal College of General Practitioners, has always staunchly supported the NHS. But in a seminal article, 'Measurement of Omission', published in the *British Medical Journal* in 1982, he called the NHS to task for doing too *few* coronary artery bypasses, hip replacements and other expensive and specialized procedures. He agrees that the United States, with its bizarre structure of incentives, does far too many of these interventions, but that does not invalidate his criticism of the British system. While it is difficult to estimate just what the right number is, for most major interventions it is a figure between the American and British levels.

Take, for example, coronary artery bypass surgery. Although Wales has very high rates of coronary disease, in the early 1980s there were only twenty bypass operations for every million people – at a time when the south-east Thames region had proportionately over *ten times* as many: 250 per million. Such an enormous gap cannot be explained by age or disease differences in the two regions. These sorts of regional inequalities have persisted in the UK, and are the subject of continued strong debate both within and outside the NHS.

What is less discussed is that in the United States the bypass rate is more than double the British average – 500 per million in the early 1980s, and many of them unnecessary and inappropriate operations. But in Sweden and Canada, where effective economic controls prevent such abuses, the rate is lower than in the US but substantially higher than in the UK – 300 per million for Sweden in the early 1980s. And in the 1990s the overall picture is likely to remain the same with regard to high-technology medicine: excess in the United States and deprivation in the UK.

It is not a coincidence that the Canadian proportion of GDP spent on health care is roughly halfway between the British and American levels – around nine per cent. Canada accomplishes less in the realms of high technology care than the US does, but that is not because it has a national health programme but because the US leaves forty million people without insurance coverage for basic health care. Britain, like Canada, has universal coverage; but because it has chosen to spend only about two-thirds of what the Canadians spend, it remains substantially behind Canada in the availability of procedures on or near the technological frontier of medicine. But both Britain and Canada have, so far, succeeded fairly well in avoiding out-of-control bureaucracy, large-volume needless surgery, malpractice-suit shenanigans and other peculiarly American problems.

'Universal coverage', however, still permits some stonewalling of disadvantaged people. Doctor Tudor Hart has spent his life dealing day-to-day with Welsh coal miners and their families. He has had to look into the eyes of many men with heart disease and tell them that they cannot get a bypass operation except after a long wait, or until they get much sicker, because the NHS simply won't give it to them. But he knows that in many cases they are already sick enough. Tudor Hart's affection and support for the NHS cannot outweigh his frustration at this unfair process of rationing; it is just not good medicine.

To an American outsider, one of the most impressive things about the British General Election of 1992 was listening to John Major talk about the NHS. Here is a man frequently compared to Ronald Reagan and George Bush – not to mention Margaret Thatcher. He is a staunch opponent of creeping socialism and even of creeping social welfare, an enemy of high taxes, a proponent of market capitalism if there ever was one. So when I saw him being interviewed about health, I was prepared for the time-worn Conservative wisdom about competition and private enterprise, freedom and privacy, leading up to a blow struck against the NHS. Instead I heard him promise faithfully that nothing would be directed towards re-establishing the privately organized medicine of half a century ago. Granted, given politics as usual, this was not a completely disingenuous statement, and there are certainly ways that the NHS can and indeed may be undermined by persistent Conservative ill will. Granted too, Major's promise may not reflect what he believes in his heart of hearts.

Nevertheless, the point I got out of it was that a newly elected Prime Minister, riding a long-rolling wave of support for Conservative economics and politics, cannot be re-elected without promising not to manhandle the NHS. This not only suggests to me that the British people love the NHS more than they dislike socialism, even now; it also suggests that the NHS, whatever its faults, is working, and working well.

The debates will undoubtedly go on, but as National Health expert Rudolf Klein put it in a February 1992 editorial in the *British Medical Journal*, 'The conflict between the two main parties is now over means not ends.' Both recognize the need for more health promotion, 'that improving health entails dealing with the social and economic conditions that cause disease and disability'. While criticizing some recent Tory reforms, Labour evidently accepts the placing of substantial economic power in the hands of general practitioners, with the aim of helping them regulate the flow of patients and money to more specialized care. But neither party has worked out how to implement the all-important reforms that will place more emphasis on maintaining health rather than curing illness.

Yet here too Britain has a tremendous advantage over the American system – one pointed out by Doctor Tudor Hart in his book, *A New Kind of Doctor* (1988). Unlike the American *or* the Canadian system, the British system does not pay doctors for piecework. Although Canadian physicians are paid by the government, while US physicians are paid by individuals, private insurers or government, both are paid for each visit to the surgery, each test, each procedure. British physicians are, in contrast, salaried by the government. If they are general practitioners, they are assigned a panel of people – usually around 2000 – and they are responsible for taking care of whatever illness comes up in those people, who only become *patients* when ill, even though the doctor is responsible for them whether they are ill or not.

Human nature being what it is, and the incentives being what they are, British physicians are likely to do too little, just as American physicians are likely to do too much. British general practitioners work very hard, and if people in their panel don't show up in the surgery, the GP is not likely to go out looking for them, which would only generate more work without generating any more money. Yet to go out looking for them may be precisely, as it were, what the doctor ordered. A recent report by the prestigious Kings Fund Centre in London recommends a new kind of medicine in which some forty per cent of London hospitals should be closed in favour of the same health cash being spent out in the community.

Studies in the UK have shown that there are many common conditions which could be readily treatable by the GPs in their surgeries – or to be more precise, in their communities. Yet less than half of men in their forties, for example, had had their blood pressure checked by their family doctor within the past ten years. In cases of death related to high blood pressure, almost half had not had their illness recognized, or had had it recognized but not treated. Many more were treated only adequately. Those who had been properly treated for this common and dangerous ailment represented only a tiny minority of those who died.

Similarly discouraging studies have been made of diabetes. In one large group practice with 20 000 patients, fifty-two per cent of all diabetics who could be identified were having no regular supervision from physicians or hospital clinics. That is a dangerous situation for a diabetic to be in. Similar statistics have been collected for asthma, chronic bronchitis and epilepsy – all serious illnesses that can be treated if identified, yet as much as half the medical care for sufferers from these disorders may be omitted.

These figures may seem alarming, but Britain has extremely good mortality and life expectancy statistics when compared with other industrial nations: the United States is far behind Britain and other countries in these key measures. Still, Britain has a far more homogeneous and health-conscious population than the US, and so could have even better mortality statistics than it does. And more important, perhaps, are the measures of health that go beyond mortality: feeling well, being vigorous and productive, being free of pain.

In October 1948 Aneurin Bevan, the inspirational founder and leader of the NHS, said, 'What we are doing is now being watched by the whole world.' More than four decades later, it is still being so watched, and it has held up very well. Bevan was not under the illusion that things would go smoothly; he also said, 'This is a very great test of the maturity of the British people.' He believed they would have to 'use this thing as though it were their own – because it is in fact their own'.

As an outsider it seems to me that the British people have passed this test of maturity – a test of a kind that my own country does not yet have the courage even to contemplate, much less rise to. In Bevan's words, 'Society becomes ... spiritually healthier if it knows that its citizens have at the back of their consciousness the knowledge that not only themselves, but all their fellows, have access, when ill, to the best that medical care can provide.' The US, in contrast, remains bogged down in an every-man-for-himself frontier mentality; thus it is not surprising that the social contract has recently broken down in Los Angeles, Atlanta and elsewhere in America, bringing back the violence as well as the philosophy of the wild frontier. America has thus proved another of Bevan's wise sayings: 'No society can legitimately call itself civilized if a sick person is denied aid because of lack of means.' That is because civilization – indeed any social contract – is based on hope and trust.

What makes hope possible, even in poverty in an advanced industrial state? Work that enables you to turn your will and energy into a decent living for you and your family. A belief that your children will have some real chance of escaping poverty. An assurance that, no matter how badly you fail, you and your children will not be allowed to be ill without aid.

Britain after the Second World War opted to make sacrifices to maintain a national health system that prevents such social fragmentation and breakdown – not to mention the guilt and shame that decent people feel at their society's neglect of and lack of compassion for those in need. I hope Britain will maintain and, to some degree, extend those sacrifices; not let them be eroded by worship of technology or illusions as to the value of private medicine; not permit the breakdown of trust between doctor and patient, between medicine and the public, that today poisons every doctor-patient encounter in the United States. Let it maintain the large corps of general practitioners, keep it strong, and place if anything more purchasing power in its hands. Let it give those dedicated, intelligent men and women enough room to breathe in their surgeries so that their youthful idealism is not steadily changed to cynical fatigue. And give them the money and time to practise the kind of medicine they know is right.

There are several things to do with this money – which, after all, would only be designed to bring Britain up to the spending level of Canada, France, Germany and other national health care systems. First, there should be a somewhat larger number of specialized procedures, such as coronary bypass and hip replacement operations, and specialized tests such as magnetic resonance imaging and echocardiograms. These techniques should be increased very judiciously – far more so than they have been in the US – taking exceptional care to prevent them from undermining, economically or psychologically, the status of GPs. Second, regional inequalities in the provision of care need to be ironed out, not by taking something away from London, but by bringing the less advantaged areas up to the level of the south-east Thames region. Third, attention should be paid to treatable chronic illness throughout the nation – a goal that can only be reached by strengthening the hand of the general practitioner.

Above all, there may be a unique opportunity to enhance the effectiveness of GPs. The same situation – responsibility for a panel of potential patients, rather than fee-for-service medicine – which holds the risk of encouraging the GP to do less intervention, can also encourage more preventive care and more outreach work. If, after all, doctors are paid the same salary regardless of how many of their 2000 (or preferably 1700) patients have heart attacks, then they can probably gain themselves more leisure time if they can reduce the number of heart attacks they have to attend to.

That means a strategy for monitoring the health of the panel of patients and reducing their risk. It means monitoring and controlling diabetes, excessive blood cholesterol, chronic obstructive lung disease and probably high blood pressure – all of which can be treated well with medicines and/or by lifestyle changes. The prevention and treatment of obesity, excess animal fat intake and, most important, smoking would greatly reduce the rate of these diseases; in turn, dismal outcomes like heart attack would be fewer and farther between. Even if the ultimate health crises were merely postponed rather than prevented, the gain in years of active, healthy life would surely be worth the trouble and cost of preventive medicine.

What is lacking is the proper training and structure in the system to facilitate health monitoring, outreach work, prevention and education. As Doctor Tudor Hart points out, the Osler paradigm of medical practice and medical education – 'Limit your horizon to a twenty-four-hour cycle' – misses a great part of what medicine can do. Equally restrictive is our inadequate notion of science. Science is not just what you do with a microscope or a genetic test; it is also a set of equations for predicting the future spread of AIDS with or without free condoms, or a statistical measurement of how many lives will be saved – or for that matter, how many pounds sterling – by identifying all the diabetics in Glyncorrwg.

Unfortunately, GPs and other physicians receive virtually no training in this kind of science – epidemiology, statistics and outcomes analysis. It is ironic that medical schools, in Britain as in the US, almost worship Rudolf Virchow for his pursuit of the under-the-microscope sort of science, but ignore completely his lifelong dedication to social medicine. The science of epidemiology – epitomized by John Snow's successful search for the water pump in Soho that was the source of so many deaths from cholera – has since advanced if anything more than under-the-microscope science. In the US, in the UK and elsewhere we need to become serious about teaching such social science in medical school.

And, of course, the art of medicine is every bit as vital in prevention as in intervention. It is the GP who is ideally situated to practise this art – to know his or her patient panel, their styles of life and work, their habits, their hopes and dreams – even their genetic ancestry. It is the GP who, like 'Doctor John' in Clifden, Ireland, can work with visiting nurses, home helps and others to stand between the patient panel and major illness. It is the GP who can decide which chronic smoker can benefit best from a stern lecture, which from a gentle ironic prod and which from a mutual belly laugh about human nature and its failings.

It has often been said that doctors cannot change human nature; but as my friend in the inner city walk-in clinic, Doctor Sally McNagny, tells her medical students, if you stop only five per cent of your smoking patients from pursuing this deadly habit, you will save more lives than by heroic intervention in the same number of patients with end-stage congestive heart failure. She knows very well that prevention is an uphill fight; but so is much else in life and in medicine. There is a Latin saying that water breaks down stone not through power but through persistence. Or in the words of the Talmud, 'It is not up to you to complete the work, but neither are you free to desist from it.'

The ancient Roman orator Cicero was not a physician, but he spoke with current relevance when he said, 'The competent physician, before he attempts to give medicine to his patient, makes himself acquainted not only with the disease which he wishes to cure, but also with the habits and constitution of the sick man.' Unfortunately this ancient wisdom has too often given way in our time to an interventionist medicine in which only curative power matters, and in which a dramatic encounter between doctor and disease, instrument and test result, by-passes almost entirely the patient, the lifestyle and the community. The challenge in Britain and other countries throughout the world is to preserve or restore the ancient balance between the two approaches, and to make medicine once again the effective, revered and noble profession which it has been for so much of the past.

REFERENCES

GENERAL BACKGROUND

Amler, Robert W. and Dull, H. Bruce, eds, *Closing the Gap: The Burden of Unnecessary Illness* (New York: Oxford University Press), 1987

Beeson, Paul, 'Changes in Medical Therapy During the Past Half Century', *Medicine 59*, pp.79–99, 1980

Callahan, Daniel, *What Kind of Life: The Limits of Medical Progress* (New York: Simon and Schuster), 1990

Carmichael, Ann G. and Ratzan, Richard M., eds, *Medicine: A Treasury of Art and Literature* (New York: Macmillan/Hugh Lauter Levin), 1991

Cassell, Eric J., *The Nature of Suffering and the Goals of Medicine* (New York: Oxford University Press), 1991

McGrew, Roderick E., *Encyclopedia of Medical History* (London: Macmillan Press), 1985

McHugh, Paul R. and Slavney, Phillip R., *The Perspectives of Psychiatry* (Baltimore: The Johns Hopkins University Press), 1983

McKeown, Thomas, *The Role of Medicine: Dream, Mirage, or Nemesis?* 2nd edn (Princeton, New Jersey: Princeton University Press), 1979

Payer, Lynn, *Medicine and Culture: Notions of Health and Sickness* (London: Victor Gollancz), 1990

Reynolds, Richard and Stone, John, eds, *On Doctoring* (New York: Simon and Schuster), 1991

Schieber, George J., Poullier, Jean-Pierre and Greenwald, Leslie M., 'Health Care Systems in Twenty-Four Countries', *Health Affairs 10*, pp.22–38, 1991

Starr, Paul, *The Social Transformation of American Medicine* (New York: Basic Books), 1982

Tudor Hart, Julian, *A New Kind of Doctor* (London: Merlin Press), 1988

White, Kerr, *The Task of Medicine: Dialogue at Wickenburg* (Menlo Park, Calif.: Kaiser Family Foundation), 1988

1 CODE OF SILENCE

Konner, Melvin, 'Transcendental Medication', *The Sciences 25*, 2–4, 1985; reprinted in Konner, *Why the Reckless Survive, and Others Secrets of Human Nature* (New York: Viking), 1989, pp.19–28

Fields, Howard L. and Levine, Jon D., 'Biology of Placebo Analgesia', *American Journal of Medicine 70*, pp.745–6, 1981

Ruberman, William et al, 'Psychosocial Influences on Mortality after Myocardial Infarction', *New England Journal of Medicine 311*, pp.552–9, 1984

Ulrich, Roger S., 'View through a Window May Influence Recovery from Surgery', *Science 224*, pp.420–1, 1984

Hippocrates, 'Decorum', excerpted in Carmichael and Ratzan, *Medicine: A Treasury of Art and Literature*, pp.36–9

Konner, Melvin, 'Laughter and Hope', *The New York Times Magazine*, 13 March 1988, pp.49–50

Cousins, Norman, *Anatomy of an Illness as Perceived by the Patient* (New York: Norton), 1979

Taylor, Shelley E., *Positive Illusions: Creative Self-Deception and the Healthy Mind* (New York: Basic Books), 1989

Cassel, Eric J., 'The Nature of Suffering and the Goals of Medicine', *New England Journal of Medicine 306*, pp.639–45, 1982

Becker, Howard S., Gear, Blanche, Hughes, Everett C. and Strauss, Anselm L., *Boys in White: Student Culture in Medical School* (Chicago: The University of Chicago), 1961

Mizrahi, Terry, *Getting Rid of Patients: Contradictions in the Socialization of Physicians* (New Brunswick, New Jersey: Rutgers University Press), 1986

Kassirer, Jerome P. and Pauker, Stephen G., 'The Toss-Up', *New England Journal 305*, pp.1467–9, 1981

Williams, Tennessee, *Cat on a Hot Tin Roof* (New York: New American Library), 1955

2 TEMPLE OF SCIENCE

Osler, William, *Aequanimitas: With Other Addresses to Medical Students, Nurses, and Practitioners of Medicine* (McGraw Hill, New York), 1932

Weissman, Gerald, 'Against Aequanimitas', *Hospital Practice*, June 1984

Tudor Hart, Julian, *A New Kind of Doctor*, op. cit.

Fletcher, David, 'Junior Doctors Win Reduction in Work Hours', *Daily Telegraph*, 17 December 1990

American College of Physicians, 'Working Conditions and Supervision for Residents in Internal Medicine Programs: Recommendations', *Annals of Internal Medicine 110*, pp.657–63, 1989

Colwill, Jack, M., 'Where Have All the Primary Care Applicants

Gone?', *New England Journal of Medicine 326*, pp.387–93, 1992; editorial by Robert G. Petersdorf, pp.408–9

Rosenberg, Charles E., *The Care of Strangers: The Rise of America's Hospital System* (New York: Basic Books), 1987

Amler and Dull, *Closing the Gap*, op. cit.

3 THE MAGIC BULLET

McGrew, Roderick, *Encyclopedia of Medical History*, op. cit.

Noller, Kenneth L., 'In Utero Exposure to Diethylstilbestrol', in Jones, Howard W. III, Wentz, Anne Colston, and Burnett, Lonnie S., *Novak's Textbook of Gynecology*, 11th edn (Baltimore, London and Sydney: Williams and Wilkins), 1988, pp.623–42

Silvestre, Louise et al, 'Voluntary Interruption of Pregnancy with Mifepristone (RU 486) and a Prostaglandin Analogue: A Large-Scale French Experience', *New England Journal of Medicine 322*, pp.625–48, 1990; editorial by Sheldon Segal, pp.691–3

Palca, Joseph and Cherfas, Jeremy, 'The Pill of Choice?', 'Etienne-Emile Baulieu: In the Eye of the Storm' and related articles, *Science 245*, pp.1319–24, 1989

Eisenberg, Leon, 'Rudolph Karl Ludwig Virchow: Where Are You Now That We Need You?', *American Journal of Medicine 77*, pp.524–32, 1984

Rosen, George, 'What Is Social Medicine?', *Bulletin of the History of Medicine 21*, pp.674–733, 1947

Troyat, Henri, *Chekhov*, trans. Michael Henry Heim (New York: Ballantine), 1986

Wolfe, Sidney M., Fugate, Lisa, Hulstrand, Elizabeth P., Kamimoto, Laurie E. et al, *Worst Pills, Best Pills: The Older Adult's Guide to Avoiding Drug-Induced Death or Illness* (Washington, DC: Public Citizen Health Research Group), 1988

Duffy, Marjorie A., et al, *Physicians' Desk Reference*, 46th edn (Montvale, New Jersey: Medical Economics Data), 1992

Wilkes, Michael S., Doblin, Bruce H. and Shapiro, Martin F., 'Pharmaceutical Advertisements in Leading Medical Journals: Experts' Assessments', *Annals of Internal Medicine 116*, pp.912–19, 1992; editorials by David A. Kessler, and Robert and Suzanne Fletcher

Chren, Mary-Margaret, Landefeld, Seth and Murray, Thomas H., 'Doctors, Drug Companies, and Gifts', *Journal of the American Medical Association 262*, pp.3448–51, 1989

Kessler, David A., 'Drug Promotion and Scientific Exchange: The

Role of the Clinical Investigator', *The New England Journal of Medicine 325*, pp.201–3, 1991

4 CONCEIVING THE FUTURE

Huxley, Aldous, *Brave New World* (New York: Bantam Books), 1946

Kevles, Daniel and Hood, Leroy, eds, *The Code of Codes: Scientific and Social Issues in the Human Genome Project* (Cambridge, Mass.: Harvard University Press), 1992

Davis, Bernard D., *The Genetic Revolution: Scientific Prospects and Public Perceptions* (Baltimore and London: The Johns Hopkins University Press), 1991

Kevles, Daniel, *In the Name of Eugenics: Genetics and the Uses of Human Heredity* (New York: Viking), 1985

Chorover, Stephan, *From Genesis to Genocide* (Cambridge, Mass.: MIT Press), 1979

Kamin, Leon, *The Science and Politics of I.Q.* (Potomac, Maryland: Lawrence Erlbaum), 1974

Associated Press, 'Health Minister Issues Warning on Hereditary Diseases, Illiteracy', Associated Press, 24 January 1990, AM Cycle

Schweisberg, David R., 'China Province Issues Sterilization Law', United Press International, 23 February 1990

Associated Press, 'Province in China Sterilizes the Retarded', *Chicago Tribune*, 22 May 1990, final edn, p.4

Goodwin, Frederick K. and Jamison, Kay Redfield, *Manic-Depressive Illness* (New York and Oxford: Oxford University Press), 1990

Jamison, Kay Redfield, Chapter 14 in Goodwin and Jamison, ibid.

Andreasen, Nancy C., 'Creativity and Mental Illness: Prevalence Rates in Writers and Their First Degree Relatives', *American Journal of Psychiatry 144,* pp.1288–92, 1987

Akiskal, Hagop S. and Akiskal, Kareen, 'Reassessing the Prevalence of Bipolar Disorders: Clinical Significance and Artistic Creativity', *Psychiatry and Psychobiology 3*, pp.29s–36s, 1988

Richards, Ruth et al, 'Creativity in Manic-Depressives, Cyclothymes, Their Normal Relatives, and Control Subjects', *Journal of Abnormal Psychology 97*, pp.281–8, 1988

Pauls, David L. and Leckman, James F., 'The Inheritance of Giles de la Tourette's Syndrome and Associated Behaviors', *The New England Journal of Medicine 315*, pp.993–7, 1986

Kurlan, Roger et al, 'Severity of Tourette's Syndrome in One Large Kindred', *Archives of Neurology 44*, pp.268–9, 1987

Wheeler, David L., 'Hunting the Tourette-Syndrome Gene: A Study in the Rigors of Scientific Detective Work', *Chronicle of Higher Education*, 23 September 1987

Kolata, Gina, 'As Fears About a Fetal Test Grow, Many Doctors Are Advising Against It', *New York Times*, 15 July 1992, p.87

Thomas, Lewis, 'The Wonderful Mistake', in *The Medusa and the Snail* (New York: Viking), 1979, pp.27–30

5 RANDOM CUTS

Wennberg, John and Gittelsohn, Alan, 'Variation in Medical Care among Small Areas', *Scientific American 246*, pp.120–34

Vayda, Eugene, Mindell, William R. and Rutkow, Ira M., 'A Decade of Surgery in Canada, England and Wales, and the United States', *Archives of Surgery 117*, pp.846–53, 1982

Vayda, Eugene and Mindell, William R., 'Variations in Operative Rates: What Do They Mean?', *Surgical Clinics of North America 62*, pp.627–39, 1982.

Chassin, M. R. et al, 'Variations in the Use of Medical and Surgical Services by the Medicare Population', *New England Journal of Medicine 314*, pp.285–90, 1986; editorial by John Wennberg, 'Which Rate is Right?', p.310

The EC/IC Bypass Group, 'Failure of Extracranial-Intracranial Arterial Bypass to Reduce the Risk of Ischemic Stroke: Results of an International Randomized Trial', *New England Journal of Medicine 313*, pp.1191–1200, 1985; follow-up article with reply to critics, *316*, pp.817–24

European Coronary Surgery Study Group, 'Long-Term Results of Prospective Randomised Study of Coronary Artery Bypass Surgery in Stable Angina Pectoris', *The Lancet 2*, pp.1173–80, 1982

Valenstein, Elliot S., *Great and Desperate Cures: The Rise and Decline of Psychosurgery and Other Radical Treatments for Mental Illness* (New York: Basic Books), 1986

Greenspan, Allan M. et al, 'Incidence of Unwarranted Implantation of Permanent Cardiac Pacemakers in a Large Medical Population', *New England Journal of Medicine 318*, pp.158–63, 1988

Ornish, Dean et al in The Lifestyle Heart Trial, 'Can Lifestyle Changes Reverse Coronary Heart Disease?', *The Lancet 336*, pp.129–33, 1990

Goleman, Daniel, 'Life-Style Shift Can Unclog Ailing Arteries, Study Finds', *New York Times*, 14 November 1989

Blakeslee, Sandra, 'Arteries Are Unblocked Without Drugs in Study', *New York Times*, 21 July 1990

6 DISORDERED STATES

Bassuk, Ellen L., 'The Homelessness Problem', *Scientific American 251*, pp.40–5, 1984

Gudeman, Jon E. and Shore, Miles F., 'Beyond Deinstitutionalization: A New Class of Facilities for the Mentally Ill', *New England Journal of Medicine 311*, pp.832–6, 1984

Mechanic, David and Aiken, Linda H., 'Improving the Care of Patients With Chronic Mental Illness', *New England Journal of Medicine 317*, pp.1634–8, 1987

Kleinman, Arthur G., *Rethinking Psychiatry: From Cultural Category to Personal Experience* (London: Collier Macmillan Publishers), 1988

Konner, Melvin, 'Anthropology and Psychiatry', in Kaplan, H. and Sadock, B., eds, *Comprehensive Textbook of Psychiatry*, 5th edn (Baltimore and London: Williams and Wilkins), 1989, pp.283–98

MacGregor, John M., *The Discovery of the Art of the Insane* (Princeton, New Jersey: Princeton University Press), 1989

Kevles, Daniel, *In the Name of Eugenics*, op. cit.

Dundes, Alan and Falassi, Alessandro, *La Terra in Piazza: An Interpretation of the Palio of Siena* (Berkeley, Calif.: University of California), 1975

Lin, Keh-Ming and Kleinman, Arthur M., 'Psychopathology and the Clinical Course of Schizophrenia: A Cross-Cultural Perspective', *Schizophrenia Bulletin 14*, pp.555–67, 1988

7 LIFE SUPPORT

Fries, James F., 'Aging, Natural Death, and the Compression of Morbidity', *New England Journal of Medicine 303*, pp.130–6, 1980

Schneider, E.L. and Brody, J.A., 'Aging, Natural Death, and the Compression of Morbidity: Another View', *New England Journal of Medicine 309*, pp.854–6, 1983

Fries, James F., 'Aging, Illness, and Health Policy: Implications of the Compression of Morbidity', *Perspectives in Biology and Medicine 31*, pp.407–28, 1988

Callahan, Daniel, *Setting Limits: Medical Goals in an Aging Society* (New York: Simon and Schuster), 1987

Homer, Paul and Holstein, Martha, eds, *A Good Old Age?: The Paradox of Setting Limits* (New York: Simon and Schuster), 1990 (Debate on Callahan's radical proposal)

Gibbs, Nancy, 'Love and Let Die', *Time*, 19 March 1990, pp.62–71 (Overview of American 'right-to-die' cases)

Wanzer, Sidney H. et al, 'The Physician's Responsibility Toward Hopelessly Ill Patients', *New England Journal of Medicine 320*, pp.844–9, 1989

Warden, John, 'Euthanasia Around the World: Britain', *British Medical Journal 304*, pp.9–10, 1992

Gomez, Carlos F., *Regulating Death: Euthanasia and the Case of the Netherlands* (New York: The Free Press), 1991

Cassel, Christine, 'The Limits of *Setting Limits,*' in Homer and Holstein, *A Good Old Age*, pp.196–206

Humphry, Derek, *Final Exit: The Practicalities of Self-Deliverance and Assisted Suicide for the Dying* (Eugene, Oregon: The Hemlock Society), 1991

Annas, George J., 'The Health Care Proxy and the Living Will', *New England Journal of Medicine 324*, pp.1210–13, 1991

8 Pandemic

Johnson, Anne M., 'Home Grown Sexually Acquired HIV Infection: Still Difficult to Predict', *British Medical Journal 304*, pp.1125–6, 1992

Mason, J.K., 'Recording HIV Status on Police Computers', *British Medical Journal 304*, pp.995–6, 1992

Brennan, Troyen A., 'Public Health Policy and the AIDS Epidemic: An End to HIV Exceptionalism?', *New England Journal of Medicine 324*, pp.1500–9, 1991; editorial by Marcia Angell, pp.1498–1500

Cowley Geoffrey, 'Tuberculosis: a Deadly Return', *Newsweek*, 16 March 1992, pp.53–7

Snider, Dixie E. and Roper, William L., 'The New Tuberculosis', *New England Journal of Medicine 326*, pp.703–5, 1992

Ford, Nicholas and Koetsawang, Suporn, 'The Socio-Cultural Context of the Transmission of HIV in Thailand', *Social Science and Medicine 33*, pp.405–14, 1991

Rhodes, Richard, 'Death in the Candy Store: The Prostitution Capital of the World, Thailand is Committing Sexual Suicide by HIV Infection', *Rolling Stone*, 28 November 1991

Clements, Alison, 'Thailand Stifles AIDS Campaign', *British Medical Journal 304*, p.1264, 1992

Mann, Jonathan, 'The New Health Care Paradigm', *Focus: A Guide to AIDS Research and Counseling 6*, pp.1–2, February 1991; adapted from a speech made in June 1990 at the Sixth International Conference on AIDS (published by the University of California, San Francisco, AIDS Health Project)

Kingman, Sharon, 'AIDS Brings Health into Focus', *New Scientist*, 20 May 1989, pp.37–42

Motivational Educational Entertainment, Research Division, *Reaching the Hip-Hop Generation* (Princeton, New Jersey: Robin Wood Johnson Foundation)

Snow, John, 'The Cholera Near Golden Square', in Carmichael and Ratzan, eds, *Medicine: A Treasury of Art and Literature*, pp.152–5

StreetwizeComicsPresent, *Gaolwize*(Sydney, New South Wales: Department of Community Services and Health Youth Rights Comics)

Lohr, Steve, 'There's No Preaching, Just the Clean Needles', *New York Times*, 29 February 1988, p.4

Trebach, Arnold S. and Zeese, Kevin B., *Drug Prohibition and the Conscience of Nations* (Washington, DC: The Drug Policy Foundation), 1990

Greer, Pedro J., Jr, 'Medical Problems of the Homeless: Consequences of Lack of Social Policy – A Local Approach', *University of Miami Law Review 45*, 407–16

Bassuk, Ellen L., 'Homeless Families', *Scientific American 265*, pp.66–74, 1991

Amler and Dull, *Closing the Gap*, op. cit.

Wachter, Robert M., 'AIDS, Activism, and the Politics of Health', *New England Journal of Medicine 326*, pp.128–32, 1992

Hacker, Andrew, *Two Nations: Black and White, Separate, Hostile, Unequal* (New York: Scribner's), 1992

Inhorn, Marcia and Brown, Peter, 'The Anthropology of Infectious Disease', *Annual Review of Anthropology 19*, pp.89–117, 1990

United Nations Children's Fund (UNICEF), *The State of the World's Children, 1990* (New York and Oxford: Oxford University Press), 1990

EPILOGUE: A NEW KIND OF DOCTOR

Allsop, Judy, *Health Policy and the National Health Service* (London: Longman), 1984 (A history, with a collection of relevant historical documents)

Tudor Hart, Julian, 'Measurement of Omission', *British Medical Journal 284*, pp.1686–9, 1982

Klein, Rudolf, 'Labour's Health Policy: The Conflict Between the Two Main Parties Is Now Over Means Not Ends', *British Medical Journal 304*, pp.517–18, 1992

Tudor Hart, Julian, *A New Kind of Doctor*, op. cit.

Tudor Hart, Julian, 'A New Type of General Practitioner', *The Lancet 2*, pp.27–9, 1983

Maxwell, Robert, 'Aneurin Bevan on the NHS', *British Medical Journal 304*, p.200, 1992

Klein, Rudolf, 'NHS Reforms: The First Six Months', *British Medical Journal 304*, pp.199–200, 1992

Kingman, Sharon, Bain, John, Smith, Jane, Whitty, Paula, Jones, Ian and Delamothe, Tony, 'The New NHS: First Year's Experience', series of 5 articles, *British Medical Journal 304*, pp.907–9; 971–3; 1036–9; 1039–41; 1109–11, 1992